Online Supervision

As online therapy becomes more mainstream, the importance of using a means of supervision which parallels this is increasingly being recognised by practitioners and the professional bodies. Very little has been written about this newly developing way of working, so this book is timely. Online Supervision: A Handbook for Practitioners covers a wide range of issues, from the practical aspects of how supervision happens, through research, legal and ethical issues to specific therapeutic settings and issues. Existing models of supervision are considered in the context of the online setting and new models which have been developed specifically for supervising online are explored.

All chapters are authored by experienced online therapists and supervisors, who bring their considerable knowledge from their practice to illuminate this growing area of the profession. In many chapters, anonymised case examples illustrate the text, alongside reflective activities which readers can choose to undertake.

While the book aims to develop the practice of online supervision of online therapists, it is recognised that there are circumstances which mean that some practitioners may choose to engage in online supervision of their face-to-face work. This is recognised and guidelines for offering and engaging in online supervision are discussed. Many practitioners begin to offer online supervision without specialised training and the final chapter centres on a discussion about the value and necessity of undertaking preparation for working in a new medium.

Online Supervision: A Handbook for Practitioners will be highly readable and accessible to both experienced practitioners and newcomers to this field.

Anne Stokes was a senior accredited BACP counsellor and a trainer, and also had a large supervision practice. She was a Director of Online Training Ltd, founding the OCTIA Conferences (Online Counselling and Therapy In Action) with her co-director, Gill Jones, and was instrumental in setting up ACTO (Association for Counselling and Therapy Online). Currently she divides her time between her homes in the UK and France, and is trying to retire! She worked at Bristol University for 15 years, leading the Diploma in Counselling at Work and the MSc in Counselling Training and Supervision, and visits Malta regularly to facilitate modules on the Masters programme on Brief Therapy and E-Counselling. Anne has written a number of books, many articles and contributed chapters. One of the enjoyable things she did recently was to work with Tim Bond to produce a number of short filmed vignettes on therapeutic issues (accessible through the 4th edition of *Standards and Ethics in Counselling in Action*). She spearheaded the BACP curricula for e-therapy training and training trainers to deliver it.

Psychotherapy 2.0 Series
Series editor: Philippa Weitz

Also in the Series

Psychotherapy 2.0
Where Psychotherapy and Technology Meet
Edited by Philippa Weitz

Online Supervision

A Handbook for Practitioners

Edited by Anne Stokes

Routledge
Taylor & Francis Group

LONDON AND NEW YORK

First published 2018
by Routledge
2 Park Square, Milton Park, Abingdon, Oxon OX14 4RN

and by Routledge
711 Third Avenue, New York, NY 10017

Routledge is an imprint of the Taylor & Francis Group, an informa business

British Library Cataloguing-in-Publication Data
A catalogue record for this book is available from the British Library

Library of Congress Cataloging-in-Publication Data
A catalog record has been requested for this book

ISBN: 9781782204794 (pbk)

Typeset in Times New Roman
by Apex CoVantage, LLC

Contents

PART IV
Training and trends   221

About the Editor and the Contributors

Kirstie Adamson initially trained as a lawyer and worked as a family law solicitor and in mental health for over fifteen years before becoming a counsellor. Kirstie now works part time privately and part time at the University of the West of England. She set up the online counselling service there in 2004 and then subsequently trained as an online supervisor and co-trained other counsellors to work online.

Kirstie has previously contributed to two publications *Therapists in Court* (BACP, 2005) and *Record Keeping and Confidentiality* (BACP, 2008). She provides regular training in working with suicide, law and the therapist, and working creatively.

Kirstie has a particular interest in working with adoption and works with many adoptive families with attachment, therapeutic parenting, and trauma. Kirstie is also a trained somatic experiencing practitioner.

Liane Collins is a director of Online Training for Counsellors and of Silverleaf Counselling. Prior to counselling she did degrees in psychology and in education, then worked as a teacher with many and varied differences in learning and processing. She is a BACP accredited counsellor, a supervisor and a tutor in online counselling and supervision. Her special interests are the autistic spectrum, ADHD and other neuro processing issues. She has over twenty-six years of experience in working with autism, has an adult son on the spectrum and is also on the spectrum herself. She trained online with Online Training for Counsellors in counselling and supervision, loves to share her enthusiasm for this platform for working with others and is committed to making counselling and supervision accessible to all.

Olivia Djouadi is a UKCP integrative psychotherapist and counsellor who also works as an online counsellor and supervisor. She is also a registered ACTO supervisor and presently teaches online counselling and supervision at Online Training for Counsellors. She trained with Online Training for Counsellors, and Birkbeck, The John Bowlby Centre, and Regents University, London. She has also taken courses in trauma and dissociative disorders with experts in the field within the UK. She continues to update her knowledge yearly with both experiential and academic courses. She learns from the experience of life. As an online counsellor, she works in the areas of chronic illness and trauma. Until recently she was the editor (special interest group editor) for a disabilities newsletter for Mensa, where she is a member. She is also an educator for Diabetes UK as well as offering education about controlling diabetes during Ramadan. She has travelled extensively and also works online with those in the UK as well as cross continental. She hopes trained online counsellors will become part of the NHS within the UK so that patients can get counselling when they need it.

Sally Evans is a certified transactional analyst and UKCP registered psychotherapist. She has an MSc (TA), and a post-graduate certificate in counselling supervision as well as being a certified cyber therapist (OTI). She is a registered ACTO practitioner. Sally has extensive experience of working with children and young people (CYP) both online (former clinical lead for Kooth.com) and offline (42nd Street, Brook Advisory). She was a member of the BACP expert reference group which drew up the counselling competences "Working at a distance". She has presented at national conferences (UKCP, BACP, ACTO) on the subject of CYP online and in particular working with CYP experiencing suicidal ideation online, for which is she is published. She is now an independent therapist, supervisor and trainer, who has, with Jan Stiff, developed a specific training on working with CYP online, as well as being a trainer with OLT.

Lalage Harries is an Integrative counsellor and supervisor, specialising in safeguarding and working with young people. She also has particular interest in cross cultural issues in counselling and the interface between anthropology and therapeutic practice She has worked in a variety of face-to-face and online settings including educational, health care and charitable organisations. Lalage currently works with Off the Record Croydon as online clinical supervisor and senior practitioner and has served as training officer for the ACTO executive committee. She also runs an independent practice online and in Cambridge, offering counselling and supervision.

Gill Jones, MA, MBACP Senior Accredited, began her counsellor training in 1990 after her youngest child was in secondary education. In 1991, she began her counsellor practice working as a volunteer counsellor for Mind in Milton Keynes. In 1993, she helped set up a group of independent counsellors who worked from the City Counselling Centre (Milton Keynes). She began her MA studies with the University of Birmingham in 1996 (completing them in 2000) and became an accredited counsellor in 1997. Her MA studies focused on the supervision and training of counsellors and psychotherapists. In 2001, she became a director of Online Training for Counsellors Ltd (which offers training to qualified therapists who wish to extend their practice online) and wrote and tutored their early courses. In 2002, she began an independent online counselling and supervision practice which still runs from her website, gjcounselling.co.uk. In 2006–2007, she initiated the discussions which culminated in the foundation of the Association for Counselling and Therapy Online (ACTO) and co-wrote *Online Counselling: A Handbook for Practitioners* with Anne Stokes. Together, they organised the first OCTIA (Online Counselling and Therapy in Action) conference in 2009. In 2015, she retired from her directorship of OLT and is in the process of retiring from online practice completely.

Babs McDonald is a BACP registered counsellor, as well as a trainer and a supervisor. She trained as an integrative counsellor but works mainly as a person-centred counsellor and supervisor. She works online and face-to-face in a Hertfordshire group practice where counselling and group-work *for all* is the practice ethos. Experiencing hearing loss herself as a two-year old, Babs is particularly interested working with the deaf and hard of hearing. She is currently learning British sign language.

Suzie Mosson is a co-director of Online Training for Counsellors Ltd, a tutor led organisation which trains counsellor and therapists to work online. She is a psychosexual and therapist, supervisor and tutor working with a face-to-face private practice in the heart of Central Scotland in addition to her online work which reaches across the globe. Suzie holds an executive role with both the Association of Counselling and Therapy Online and OCTIA Ltd (the annual online conference) and is chair of the Scottish Association of Psychodynamic Counselling.

Maria O'Brien is an accredited therapist with the British Association of Counselling and Psychotherapy, a member of the Association for Counselling and Therapy Online, and a director of Online Training for Counsellors Ltd (www. onlinetrainingforcounsellors.com). She originates from a small village in southern Ireland and moved to England in the late 1980s and currently resides in Hampshire.

Chris O'Mahony has worked in online mental health since 2008, focusing on widening access to emotional support and working therapeutically across cultures. Chris has worked as an online counsellor and supervisor in her native Ireland, Wales, Germany, and England, and has developed online therapy services in the charity sector. She was co-tutor on the CPCAB-accredited OLT diploma in online therapeutic supervision. Chris is completing a professional doctorate in clinical psychology at the University of East London, and works in the NHS with individuals and families experiencing severe emotional distress. She has a specialist interest in health apps, digital health, online service provision and online therapeutic relationships.

Stephanie Palin has worked in the therapy field for over thirty years, as a therapist with Relate, the NHS, and in private practice. She has been training counsellors and psychosexual therapists since 1990, and currently lectures in PST at Doncaster, working with couples, sex addiction and working online in Manchester and Edinburgh. Stephanie is a past president of the International

Society for Mental Health Online and was chair of the Association for Counselling Therapy Online. She is currently a trustee at ATSAC (Association for the Treatment of Sex Addiction and Compulsivity). She has taken part in TV and radio programmes, and was the relationship and sex expert for ManMOT, an online GP Surgery supported by Pfizer. Stephanie also acts as clinical supervisor with a group of relationship and sex therapists who work with military families in western Europe, using online resources to assist this valuable work. Stephanie's interest in digital technological influences on our lives has led her to combine her work in the sexual field with her research into the use of online pornography and its effects on relationships. Her MA dissertation (2006) explored the therapeutic relationship in online therapy.

Jan Stiff's initial career path began in Paediatric nursing, specialising in paediatric oncology and palliative care. Nursing as a palliative care nurse at Naomi House Children's Hospice, her career path took a change in direction. Jan established an in-house sibling support service to meet the emotional needs of siblings both pre- and post-bereavement. This saw the start of a passion and career in counselling children and young people. Jan has continued to be interested in the emotional needs and mental health needs of children and young people, counselling online for COAP (Children of Addicted Parents and People) and for Swings & Smiles (a charity providing recreational facilities and services for families with special needs). Jan works privately as an online supervisor and has provided online supervision for online counsellors at BeatBullying and currently for TIC+ in Gloucester (online service). Since training with Online Training for Counsellors (OLT), Jan presently works as an OLT tutor, primarily for DOTS (Diploma in Online Therapeutic Supervision). In partnership with Sally Evans (also an OLT tutor), Jan has formulated and tutored a training programme specific to the needs of CYP face-to-face counselling services, wishing to extend their services to delivering online counselling for children and young people. Jan is now membership director for ACTO (www.acto-org.uk)

Anne Stokes was a senior accredited BACP counsellor and a trainer, and also had a large supervision practice. She was a director of Online Training Ltd, founding the OCTIA conferences with her co-director, Gill Jones, and was instrumental in setting up ACTO Currently she divides her time between her homes in the UK and her home in France, and is trying to retire! She worked at Bristol University for fifteen years, leading the diploma in counselling at work and the MSc in counselling training and supervision, and visits Malta regularly to facilitate modules on the masters' programme on brief therapy and e-counselling. Anne has written a number of books, many articles, and contributed chapters. One of the enjoyable things she did recently was to work with Tim Bond to produce a number of short filmed vignettes on therapeutic issues (accessible through the 4th edition of *Standards and Ethics for Counselling in Action*). She spearheaded the BACP curricula for e-therapy training and training trainers to deliver it.

Philippa Weitz works and writes widely around counselling and psychotherapy online. She has special interests in both the success of the online therapeutic relationship, and security, confidentiality, and jurisdiction. She is a qualified teacher, trainer, and psychological counsellor with more than twenty-five years in the mental health sector. She is currently training director for The Academy for Online Counselling and Psychotherapy, director of psychotherapy services for "Dr Julian Mental Health" app, director of UK Counselling Online She is one of the professionals advising the Private Practice Hub's online therapy section, and is standards and ethics officer for ACTO. She is author/editor of *Psychotherapy 2.0: Where Psychotherapy and Technology Meet* as well as series editor for the Karnac *Psychotherapy 2.0* series. She is currently planning her next publication: *Psychotherapy 2.0: It's all About the Online Relationship.*

Acknowledgements

Like the first volume in this series, this book is very much a team effort. My thanks go to Pippa Weitz – I think! – for prodding me into finally agreeing to edit this book, after years of colleagues saying I should do so. Mainly it has been fun working with my co-authors, and felt very fitting to have had this opportunity to collaborate closely for one last time as I retired from Online Training for Counsellors Ltd. Every contributor has had some connection with OLT, as students, tutors, supervisors or advisors.

Jane Hallett is really responsible for this book, as it was she, some eighteen years ago, who asked if I would volunteer to be an online client for the nascent training organisation. If it hadn't been for her, I would have probably stayed with face-to-face work for all of my professional life. Later, after my initial online training, Gill Jones had the faith in me to ask me to become a tutor and then a co-director in OLT, so she bears some responsibility too!

My particular gratitude goes to Kirstie Adamson and Chris O'Mahony. They stayed with me at every step of the last weeks of finalising the manuscript. Kirstie has an eagle eye for split infinitives, amongst other things, as she proofreads, and Chris performed the mammoth task of checking every reference, even on Christmas Eve and Boxing Day. Most of all, my thanks to them for the wonderfully supportive emails which eased me in my most despondent hours. Despite all their help, the responsibility for any errors that remain is mine alone.

Finally, I want to acknowledge the importance of the love and patience of my husband, Jonathan. Maybe this time I will keep my promise to him to retire. Who knows!

Series Editor's Foreword

Back in the dark ages in 1987, in my first year as a qualified psychotherapist, I chose a supervisor who was as eminent as they come, an elderly analyst with many years of experience. I chose him because he had a brilliant reputation and felt lucky to have found him. It was a disaster. We simply didn't click, whatever that means (the subject of this book, of course, within the online context). The experience left me with having learned to be a bad supervisee, and being far more knowledgeable about what supervision shouldn't be, though I didn't work this out until much later.

My second (and brilliant) supervisor taught me what supervision was really about. *And we clicked.* From her I learned the passion that is involved in working with clients, the on-going quest for self-development and questioning all that I do and am as a therapist, the importance of how to use the self as part of the therapeutic alliance, and how we learn and develop through our work with our clients. She also taught me also the delights of live supervision. Our clients have so much to teach us and we need to endlessly be self-challenging about what we are doing with them. For me supervision (in whatever context) provides us with this space for reflection and growth and an opportunity to think outside the box. Carl Roger's (1973) 1972 address to the American Psychological Association, "Some new challenges", is for me the most profound article I have recently read, and it finishes with the three short words: "*Do we dare?*"

In online work, both as a supervisor and a therapist, I remain convinced that this question is fundamental to the development of the online counselling and psychotherapy, and alongside online supervision; remaining open to all the new potential of working online whilst being mindful of the pitfalls along the way. Both are covered fully within this publication.

I was privileged to be in Anne Stokes' final diploma in online therapeutic supervision cohort before she retired. Gosh, it was tough going, I had no idea I knew so little about supervision (despite thirty years in the profession as a therapist), and what I could tell you about online supervision, I could have written on a postage stamp. I had simply been uninquisitive about supervision for all those years, merely seeing as an obligatory chore to be completed.

But the diploma in therapeutic online supervision really woke me up, and took me back to what I learned from my second supervisor, who provides such excellent role modelling for being a supervisor. From Anne and her team, we learned so much on what and how online supervision can be so enhancing for the supervisee. And now you get the opportunity to share in the fruits of all this group learning. To return to my opening point about "clicking", what really interests me is the "clicking" of the supervisee and supervisor, the supervisory alliance at work, and in the context of working online, redefining and finding new ways of delivering supervision through digital methods for the benefit of all, supervisor, supervisee, and client.

This book is loaded with fascinating new models for online supervision, discussions about research and guidelines, issues of jurisdiction and risk management, including internationally, and legal and ethics considerations, as well as how online supervision opens up access to groups who might find face-to-face supervision impossible or too challenging.

As I wrote my chapter for the book, on guidelines for online supervision and supervision online, I became aware of something very important: this book is relevant to many therapists, as these days, many face-to-face therapists receive their supervision online. This book is therefore for all those face-to-face therapists and their online supervisors, and is not just a book for the specialist online therapist and supervisor. Psychotherapy went digital a long time ago (after all even Freud used the telephone) – and our clients are largely embedded in digital technology ranging from Facebook to a smart phone and all points in between – which means we must engage digitally whether we like it or not. Along with this, supervision, online and face-to-face, has gone digital too. A read of Chalfont and Pollecoff's (2014) chapter, "Challenges and dilemmas in the online consulting room" in volume 1 of *Psychotherapy 2.0* (Weitz, 2014) provides a fascinating insight to the impact "digital" has on the consulting room. No one is exempt.

I hope you'll really enjoy this second volume in the Psychotherapy 2.0 series. There are more to come! As I suggested with volume 1, it's a book to dip into, and come back to.

I thank Anne for her achievement of pulling this book together. It is team work with colleagues and former students from the diploma in online supervision and I believe this book will provide a really useful resource for therapists, supervisors, and trainers – both online and face-to-face.

Philippa Weitz
Series Editor

References

Chalfont, A. & Pollecoff, M. (2014). Challenges and dilemmas in the online consulting room. In: Weitz, P. (Ed.) (2014), *Psychotherapy 2.0: Where Psychotherapy and Technology Meet* (pp. 89–101). London: Karnac.

Rogers, C. (1973). Some new challenges. *American Psychologist*, May 1973: 379–287.

Introduction

Anne Stokes

Welcome to the book, whether you are an experienced online supervisor, an online therapist who might consider working as an online supervisor, a face-to-face therapist who receives supervision online or someone who is simply interested in knowing more. My guess is that if you own this book, you probably do already have an interest, but you could be just browsing the books on a bookstall at a CPD event and be very sceptical. You too are welcome as that is where I began my own online journey some seventeen years ago!

I am grateful to Suzie Mosson for allowing me to use, and slightly adapt, the opening lines to one of her essays. She wrote:

> Similar to Professor Jackie Kay (2016) this book hopes to "open up the conversations, the blethers, the arguments and celebrations". The future of online supervision is an ongoing learning process and this is not the end of the road.

I think she summed it up beautifully and succinctly.

The book grew out of many conversations where colleagues kept saying, "Why don't you write a book about online supervision? You've written plenty of short articles and some chapters about it." Having resisted for as long as possible, I realised that if I didn't do it now, on the brink of trying to retire, I probably never would.

My next thought was that I would prefer an edited book as these same colleagues have expertise and specialist knowledge in many areas of online supervision. Also, I have gained much from them in my own online supervision practice and particularly when I was developing the diploma in online therapeutic supervision (DOTS) for Online Training Ltd (www.onlinetrainingforcounsellors.com) and its continuing evolution.

An edited book allows for different perspectives and different voices. I have not edited out any statements where I might see things differently and I hope that the editing process has still enabled individual voices to be heard. You will discover that there are conflicting opinions between authors in some cases and I think that is healthy. It has been a real privilege working with so many talented online supervisors who are passionate about their work and prepared to share it with others.

The book is divided into sections. In Part I, I provide an outline of online supervision. This continues with an overview of the research and then looks at models old and new, as well as relationships in online supervision. Part II considers legal, ethical, regulatory, and cross-cultural issues arising when practising as an online supervisor. Specific contexts are explored in Part III. Finally, Part IV is a discussion chapter between six practitioners, focusing on training for online supervision and, very briefly, on how we see online supervision developing. As one would expect from ethical practitioners, all examples of practice within the chapters have either been fictionalised or anonymised.

There is inevitably an overlap between chapters. I make no apologies for this as it demonstrates the fundamental importance of some aspects of online supervision. Sometimes this overlap is noted, so you can follow up a theme. At other times, you will make the connection yourself as you read different chapters.

There is also a considerable variation in the length of chapters. This is partly due to the subject matter of the chapter, but also importantly because it reflects the contributors' individual styles and voices. Just as there are many differences in the styles and voices of online supervisors, it felt right to not edit out those differences here. Jane Speedy, a much-loved colleague at the University of Bristol, used to use the expression, "having the plumbing on the outside". We were particularly training counselling trainers and supervisors at MSc level, and we wanted them to understand why we were working with them in specific ways – thus they could see the plumbing! You may notice some of the washers and pipes in this book too.

It is not a book to be read in one sitting, or even from front to back. Choose the chapters that interest you and which may link back or forward to another one. There are reflective activities in many chapters which have been designed to enable you to consolidate your thinking, if you so choose. Above all, I hope that you will enjoy reading the book and find it useful.

References

Brooks, L. (2016). Jackie Kay named as new Scottish makar. *The Guardian*, 15 March 2016. Available at: www.theguardian.com/books/2016/mar/15/jackie-kay-becomes-the-new-makar-scotlands-national-poet. Accessed 25th March 2016.

Mosson, S. (2016). A description and critical analysis of my supervision model. Unpublished manuscript.

Part I

Online supervision
in practice

Chapter 1

A brief overview of online supervision

Anne Stokes

Working at a distance is not new. Freud worked with some of his patients by letter, and also discussed cases with his colleagues by mail. This has some parallels with email counselling and supervision. However, perhaps it would help to begin by stating how I use the term online supervision. My working definition is that it is supervision which comes about via use of technology of either or both face-to-face (f2f) and online therapy. So, the one thread that runs through all online supervision is about what it is not! It is not supervision which takes place with the supervisor and the supervisee(s) in the same physical space at the same time.

Speyer and Yaphe (2016) state that it is intended to "assure the quality of online counselling and effectiveness of therapeutic outcomes". They also mention the educational or formative role within online supervision to aid the supervisees in their online development. Given the paragraph above, it may also serve to enhance the quality and effectiveness of f2f therapy.

As you will read in many of the chapters which follow, online supervision may happen in a number of ways. It can occur in real-time (synchronously) or asynchronously, where the response will not be immediate. Smartphones, tablets, laptops, desktops – almost any device capable of connecting with another through the use of the internet – have been used for online supervision. It can also be one-to-one or group supervision. There are advantages and disadvantages in using all of these. Chapters two and eight in particular expand many of the points made in this brief overview, and therefore they are not detailed here to void over-repetition. Here I concentrate solely on describing how online supervision happens and do not home in on the issues surrounding the various modes in any detail.

Much of what is written by the authors in this book could also apply to telephone supervision. Indeed, the BACP's training curriculum is for telephone and e-counselling rather than solely online therapy (Stokes, 2016a).

Before looking at the delivery options, let's consider some of the reasons that therapists and supervisors might consider this way of working.

- It may parallel the manner in which the therapy is being delivered by the supervisee.
- It enables supervisees to choose from a range of supervisors who are not geographically near to them.

- If there is a specific issue which needs input from a supervisor with an expertise in a particular field, it may be easier to find and work with them.
- It may ease the issue of dual relationships in small communities where every therapist knows and is known by all others.
- Supervisees with a disability may be able to access supervision more readily – the same applies to supervisors seeking supervisees.
- While the amount of supervision required and its resulting cost per session will not be reduced, travelling time is eliminated and therefore also some cost.
- If working asynchronously, there is more flexibility in when the supervisor and the supervisee allocate their supervision time, as they will not need to be together online in real time.
- In many cases, there will be a complete record of the supervision, thus enabling reflection after and between sessions on what has been discussed.

You can probably add to this list.

It may seem that I believe that online supervision is the most effective mode of delivery for every supervisor and every supervisee. This is not where I stand. In my opinion, and indeed as suggested in Bond's (2015a) guidance for online working, where possible at least some of the supervision should be delivered by the same means as the therapy. This helps to shine the light on blind spots, parallel processes, transference etc. So, while I strongly advocate that all online therapists should have some online supervision, the reverse is true. F2f therapist should whenever possible have some f2f supervision. The insertion of "whenever possible" recognises the reality that there could be circumstances where it is not possible, but this should not happen simply for convenience.

It may be tempting for a therapist who works both f2f and online to have one supervisor who supervises both types of client work. This is convenient and often an online therapist may have already developed a very strong working relationship with their f2f supervisor, particularly if they have very few online clients. However, does the supervisor also have online clients? Are they trained as online therapists (as hopefully their supervisee will be)? Do they understand the therapeutic and technological issues that arise in online work? Do they have prejudices about f2f work being "better" or "deeper" than online therapy? Are they trained as online supervisors?

Weitz, in chapter twelve, highlights the low number of supervisors who are currently trained to offer online supervision, so this last point can cause some difficulties. Indeed, the first cohort of the diploma in online therapeutic supervision which I devised and ran, was as recent as 2013. Hopefully over the next few years, this will become less of an issue. Before becoming too obsessed by this difficulty though, we would do well to remember that in the early days of f2f counselling, a) there was no supervision and b) even when it was recognised as beneficial, it was simply provided by more experienced therapists. Only comparatively recently (in the last couple of decades) have there been plenty of trained f2f supervisors to choose from. One way round the dilemma of needing two supervisors to cover both methods of delivering therapy is discussed by Adamson in chapter eighteen.

So how does it actually happen?

If you are an online therapist, you may want to skim read this section as much of it will be familiar to you from your practice with clients! In her chapter on reflective writing (chapter eight), Jones gives case examples of the various ways of working together in supervision so they are merely explained below. There are also further case examples in Jones and Stokes (2009), and Stokes (2016b).

First, there is a need to add extras to the contract that would normally be made in f2f supervision. These include how technology difficulties will be managed; the security of the devices both parties are using; storage of data; the private nature of the working environments of both supervisor and supervisee; what the time lapses between receipt and response to emails will be, if working asynchronously; emergency contact since supervisors don't live on their computers and phones twenty-four hours a day (or shouldn't do!), and in some cases there may need to be discussion around the issues of working across national boundaries (see also chapter eleven). Even if working synchronously, it is good practice to have a written contract for online supervision which is signed by both parties. With asynchronous supervision, it is essential.

Anecdotal evidence suggests that sometimes supervisors and supervisees rush to "get on with the supervision" before talking or writing about the things that would normally be explored in an introductory session when working f2f. It is still necessary to exchange information about training, models of therapy and supervision, expectations of each other, ways of working together, range of clients and issues the supervisee works with, and particular wants or needs. Rather in the way that disinhibition may cause an online client to plunge straight in to the work without establishing who is who in the relationship, the same can happen in online supervision. Maybe this doesn't always matter, but too often it can cause problems later because of basics which have not been shared.

Email supervision

This was probably the very earliest way of providing online supervision. Supervisees may prefer to write as they reflect following a client session and find it more difficult to go back to thoughts and feelings at a later stage in a pre-booked synchronous session. Vernmark ("Depression therapy by email", 2005) found this to be so in his research into email counselling. In some online supervision contracts, the supervisor may be prepared to receive emails whenever the supervisee wishes to send them. This can work if there is a clear understanding about the amount of time within which a response will be written, as well as an agreement about how the amount of supervision required by professional bodies will be monitored by both supervisor and supervisee. Other contracts may stipulate when emails will be sent and responded to.

One of the benefits of working this way is that the supervisor has time to reflect in depth before responding to the supervision email. Another is the advantage for the supervisee in discovering that the very act of writing the email, and perhaps re-reading it, enables them to arrive at a greater or different understanding of the issue, the client or the process.

I find it useful for supervisees also to send a separate document with their supervision email, which keeps me abreast of who they are working with and a very brief overview of the current work. As with all online work, whether for therapy or supervision, emails should be encrypted and documents password protected. While no system can be guaranteed to be totally confidential, this does at least minimise the risks. I also prefer the supervision process to take place within a document, which is attached to a covering email, rather than be in the body of the email, as, if these are sent according to the protocols just mentioned, it gives a further layer of protection and security. Some may feel this is overkill.

Email supervision is also useful for emergency contact, providing the supervisor is prepared to access their inbox very regularly. It is no use setting up this possibility and then the supervisor only reading emails every couple of days. Emergencies need more immediate responses.

There are disadvantages of this method of supervision. Emails do occasionally go astray or land in junk mail, so both parties need to be attentive to sending a brief message to acknowledge their receipt. There must be agreement about what is the best way to respond to each other in practical terms such as writing within each other's email or writing in a new email (see chapter eight for examples). Length of emails, both too short and too long short, can cause problems. Sometimes style of writing by the supervisor may come over as too questioning and even unsupportive, or too woolly and equally unsupportive. It is therefore self-evident that these things need to be checked out.

Care must to be taken with the storage of supervision emails. This isn't a disadvantage, simply a reminder of the need to think through this carefully. However, actually having the ability at a later date to go back to a full record of the supervision at a particular time of a particular client may well be a great advantage.

Very occasionally, email supervision could be a way of a supervisee avoiding the perceived rigours and demands of synchronous work. While this doesn't happen often, an online supervisor should keep this in mind as a possibility, particularly if there seems to be a difficulty within the supervision working alliance.

If the supervisee works mainly by email with clients, this may well be the most appropriate method for online supervision. If, on the other hand, most of the client work is synchronous, then a parallel way of supervising should be explored.

Synchronous online supervision

There are three ways of working synchronously – text, voice, and webcam plus voice. Supervisors can use existing platforms (such as VSee) or a provision in their own websites. However, while this latter may have advantages of apparent professionalism and security, unless working within an organisation with an IT department, this is likely to be a costly option and not for the less technically literate or competent supervisors (Stokes 2016b).

Text

This is probably the most reliable technologically of the three, since it is less complex than the other two. It gives the same advantage of a record of the whole session found in supervision by email, without the disadvantage of having to wait for an email reply. Spontaneity can be much greater and some practitioners have told me that they feel that it enables the working alliance to develop more quickly. Misunderstandings which can arise in any text based work can be sorted out more speedily as there may be more immediacy in the dialogue.

However, there are also disadvantages. Perhaps the main one is the speed of typing of each participant. If one person is very slow, then there can be a sense of disconnection and the speedier person s mind may wander. It is therefore important to "just type" and to try to forget the possibility of "typos" which show up as spelling mistakes. Unless those make the words unable to be understood, it doesn't usually matter. There are other ways of speeding things up such as sending text in small amounts but indicating that there is more to come (usually using ".."). This keeps the receiver engaged. It may not be the best form of online supervision for those with dyslexia or similar language based disabilities.

Voice alone

Telephone supervision has long been widely accepted and VoIP (Voice over Internet Protocol) is very similar. So why choose an online way of supervising over using the telephone? A basic reason may be cost! VoIP is usually free, whereas even "free calls" by telephone are actually costing in some way within a package. Another reason of more interest to online supervisors and supervisees is that using a voice connection through the internet is generally more secure than using a landline and in particular, certainly more secure than using a mobile phone. A disadvantage which occurs occasionally is a delay between speaking and receiving, so that the conversation has the staccato quality which used to be a feature of international phone calls decades ago.

Often this is an effective way in to starting online supervision, as long as one thinks carefully about security and privacy. It has a security of the familiar, without that false sense of familiarity which is discussed below with webcam and voice.

Using voice and webcam together

Increasingly supervisors and supervisees are turning to using webcams for live supervision. It perhaps has the most advantages and the most disadvantages for supervision in terms of technology.

It is useful to be able to work in a way in which supervisor and supervisee can see and hear each other as it may help to increase focus, the working alliance, and intimacy. It is possible to work together on a whiteboard to draw and write; video clips, documents, and photographs can be instantly shared (well, nearly instantly depending on the speed of the connection!). It can be used for group supervision with possibly less chance of people "talking" (writing) over each other than in live text. It is an exciting way of working where change of mood and pace are easier to note and explore. There are no issues of delay due to typing speeds in live text or responses to emails. So, it can seem an easier mode to use when moving from f2f supervision. What is there not to like?

In an earlier book, I wrote about the use of webcams: "In a few years, it is possible that online supervision will be no different from f2f supervision, apart from the physical location of the participants" (Stokes, 2009, p. 109). How I regret those words! Yes, the technology has vastly improved in those eight years, and is much more reliable. However, what I failed to take in to consideration is the fact that it *is* solely face-to-face in most cases. That is to say, you cannot see the whole person, only their head and shoulders. You do not have all the visual cues you have when sitting in the same room. You do not know whether the heightened or reduced colour of someone's face is related to their emotional state or to technology. And despite being so much more reliable, both sound and picture can distort at times, which is disruptive. So, I do see webcam supervision as still being rather different to f2f and get quite antsy when I hear someone saying, "I just do a bit of skype supervision so don't need training."

That sentence also raises one of the current main bones of contention in the world of online therapy and online supervision – Skype itself. If you are working in the USA, using Skype is a definite no-no. It is not HIPAA compliant (Health Insurance Portability and Accountability Act of 1996) and will put you into an unethical and probably illegal situation. Within England, several online therapists and supervisors have sought guidance from the Information Commissioner's Office, which is responsible for the enforcement of the Data Protection Act 1998, and have received conflicting opinions. There are plenty of other available platforms to use and you would be well advised to research them (see also Weitz, chapter twelve). However, there are still many supervisees (and clients) who, even though the possible security and confidentiality issues have been thoroughly explored, will make the informed choice to remain with Skype because they are used to using it. They may well state that no platform can claim to be totally secure and confidential. Bond (2015b) highlights the strong ethical requirement to make certain that their online practice is managed competently and with sufficient security to meet their clients' needs and their professional ethical requirements. We could substitute the word "supervisees" for clients.

Conclusion

This short chapter has outlined the practicalities of the various ways in which online supervision can take place. The following chapters will flesh out how it is used practically, in various settings and some of the issues which practitioners must take into consideration when working in this medium.

Reflective questions

- Which method(s) of online supervision most attracts you? Consider the reasons for your answer.
- Which method(s) least attracts you? Again, what are the reasons for this?
- As you look at your reasons, would you be able to sustain them if discussing online supervision with a colleague?
- Are your choices the same when you think about yourself as a supervisee and then as a supervisor?
- Does this reflection highlight anything you need to discuss with your current supervisor?

References

Bond, T. (2015a). *Good Practice in Action 047: Ethical Framework for the Counselling Professions Supplementary Guidance. Working Online.* Lutterworth: BACP.

Bond, T. (2015b). *Standards and Ethics for Counselling in Action (4th edn).* London: Sage, p. 193.

Congress, US (1996, August). Health Insurance Portability and Accountability Act of 1996 (HIPAA). In: *104th US Congress. HR* (Vol. 3103, pp. 104–191).

Depression therapy by email. (2005). Theage.com.au. Available at: www.theage.com. au/news/breaking/depression-therapy-by-email/2005/08/15/1123957976731.html. Accessed 22nd December 2016.

Great Britain (1998). The Data Protection Act. London: Stationery Office.

Jones, G. & Stokes, A. (2009). *Online Counselling: A Handbook for Practitioners.* Basingstoke: Palgrave Macmillan.

Speyer, C. & Yaphe, J. (2016). An approach to the training and supervision of online counsellors. In: S. Goss, K. Anthony, L. S. Stretch, & D. M. Nagel, (Eds.), *Technology in Mental Health: Applications in Practice, Supervision and Training (2nd edn)* (p. 231). Springfield, IL: Thomas.

Stokes, A. (2016a). *Telephone and E-Counselling Training Curriculum.* Lutterworth: BACP.

Stokes, A. (2016b) Supervision in private practice. In: S. Goss, K. Anthony, L. S. Stretch, & D. M. Nagel, (Eds.), *Technology in Mental Health: Applications in Practice, Supervision and Training (2nd edn)* (pp. 331–337). Springfield, IL: Thomas.

Chapter 2

Learning from the past and looking to the future: research on online supervision

Chris O'Mahony

Introduction

Online counselling is a rapidly expanding area of counselling and psychotherapy practice and the subject of a growing body of research. Online supervision – that is, supervision that is conducted via the internet through email, live text chat, voice or video – has received far less attention. In this chapter, I examine the research to date on online supervision of online counsellors, explore what we can infer from research on related areas, and highlight what we may take from the literature to inform our own online supervision practice.

Many sections of this chapter are followed by reflective questions, which are designed to give the reader space to consider how the research could be relevant to their own work.

Reflective questions

- What aspects of in-person supervision may map over to online supervision?
- What aspects of online counselling may map over to online supervision?
- What is your personal attitude towards online supervision?

What is supervision?

It has been argued that supervision is the most important activity for the development of therapeutic competence (Ladany & Inman, 2012). Supervision has been described as:

> An intervention provided by a more senior member of a profession to a more junior member or members of the same profession. This relationship is evaluative, extends over time, and has the simultaneous purposes of enhancing the

professional functioning of the more junior person(s), monitoring the quality of professional services offered to clients [...] [serving] as a gatekeeper for those who are to enter the particular profession. (Bernard & Goodyear, 2009, p. 8)

Supervision is complementary to but distinct from training. According to Pilling and Roth (2014), *training* conveys the knowledge required to apply an intervention with clients in general, while *supervision* helps the supervisee to apply the knowledge gained in training to specific contexts and clients. For example, a student can be trained in how to use psychodynamic psychotherapy but it is in supervision that she will explore the experience of working with a client, reflect upon her practice and plan future actions. Her supervisor can offer her support and advice, and can check that the student is acting ethically in her work with the client.

There is convincing evidence that supervision is important for the wellbeing of both counsellors and clients. A strong supervisory alliance is associated with supervisees feeling more confident, more passionate about their work and more competent (Bernard & Goodyear, 2014; Goodyear & Bernard, 1998). Supervision also has more tangible effects – clinical supervision has been found to enhance the therapeutic alliance between counsellor and client, and to contribute to clients' progress (Bambling, King, Raue, Schweitzer, & Lambert, 2006; Callahan, Almstrom, Swift, Borja, & Heath, 2009). Given the many benefits of supervision for both supervisees and clients, it is unsurprising that the majority of the professional and regulatory bodies for counsellors in the UK either require or strongly recommend their qualified members to take part in ongoing supervision (e.g., BABCP, 2016; BACP, 2016; BPC, 2011; BPS, 2009; UKCP, 2012).

What is online supervision?

As mentioned in chapter one, text-based therapy and supervision work dates back to Freud, who wrote letters to his colleagues discussing clinical cases (Gay, 1998), and audio recording of sessions for supervision goes back at least as far as Rogers (Jencius, Baltimore, & Getz, 2010). More recently, telephone supervision has been used to discuss supervision sessions recorded on VHS tapes and sent in the post (Wetschler, Trepper, McCollum, & Nelson, 1993), showing that distance need not be a barrier to supervision of counselling work. Today, the term online supervision can be used to refer to a wide range of services. "Online" in this context has been used to mean any interactions facilitated by technology where the people involved are not in the same room – telephone, videoconferencing software, live text chat, email, avatar, and more. The term online supervision is also used to refer to some live supervision methods, such as "bug-in-the-ear" or "bug-in-the-eye" supervision, where the supervisor watches the supervisee in session from behind a one-way mirror and gives feedback to the supervisee via a wireless earpiece or via a computer screen.

The term online supervision has been applied to online supervision of online counselling, to online supervision of in-person counselling, or even in-person supervision of online counselling. Muddying the waters further, the word supervision has different connotations in different cultures. In North America, supervision often refers exclusively to work between a qualified professional and a trainee, whereas when two qualified professionals work together it is more commonly called consultation.

In this chapter, I have chosen to focus on online supervision (delivered via email, live text, chat, voice or video) of the online work of qualified professional counsellors, rather than online supervision of trainee counsellors.

Reflective questions

- Would you consider Freud's supervision via letter to be comparable to today's online supervision? Why or why not?

Why is online supervision important?

Reindl, Engelhardt, and Zauter (2015) conducted a study designed to take stock of the current state of online supervision in their native Germany and in the UK. The authors conducted interviews with experts in online supervision and sent a survey to members of their professional organisation, the German Association for Systemic Therapy, Counselling and Family Therapy (DGSF).

They found that online supervision was a marginal practice in Germany, and most supervision of online counselling happened in-person. Other authors caution against in-person supervision of online work, arguing that it is important that the supervision occur in the same modality as the counselling that is being reflected upon (Jones & Stokes, 2009; Reindl, 2015). An in-person supervisor may not have expertise in online communication and so may not be able to provide effective supervision of online work. Supervision in the same medium as the counselling can also make it easier to spot parallel process – that is, the mirroring in the supervision session of the process between counsellor and client (Gilbert & Evans, 2000, p. 105).

Reviewing the literature

Looking at how in-person supervision has evolved since its inception, we can see that developments in supervision tend to parallel and follow earlier developments in counselling (Bernard & Goodyear, 2004; Clingerman & Bernard, 2004; Leddick & Bernard, 1980). Online counselling is a new and developing field, and online supervision of online work has not yet been studied in depth.

There are very few published studies on online supervision of online counsellors. In reviewing the literature, I found that each of the currently available studies that are applicable to online supervision fell into one of the following categories:

1. Online supervision of qualified counsellors working online
2. Online supervision of trainee counsellors working online
3. Online supervision of qualified counsellors working in-person
4. Online supervision of trainee counsellors working in-person
5. In-person supervision of qualified counsellors working online
6. In-person supervision of trainee counsellors working online
7. In-person supervision of qualified counsellors working in-person

Most of the literature that may be categorised as online supervision falls into category four, online supervision of trainee counsellors working in-person. Fewer studies are available from categories two and three (online supervision of trainee counsellors working online and online supervision of qualified counsellors working in-person), and fewer still in category one, online supervision of qualified counsellors working online.

Although the published literature on online supervision of online counselling (category one above) is scant, I believe we can learn from adjacent areas of research. For example, online supervision of counsellors working in-person may

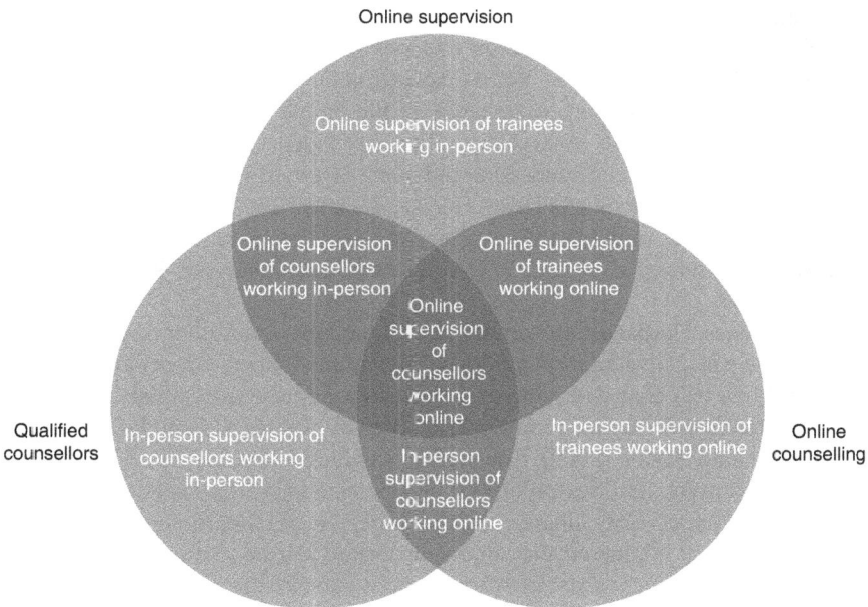

Figure 2.1 Research on online supervision

provide information on the process of online supervision, the interaction and the relationship between supervisor and supervisee. Similarly, online supervision of trainees working online may indicate how parallel process between counselling and supervision is expressed in online work.

In reviewing the literature, I have prioritised the papers examining online supervision of counsellors and trainees working online, as these are most relevant to the type of online supervision described in this book. I have then used papers examining online supervision of in-person counselling where I felt the research added to our understanding of online supervision overall.

Many of the studies cited in this chapter come from not just counselling, psychotherapy, and psychology, but also from speech and language therapy, nursing, and psychiatry. The majority of papers cited are research-based, but I also draw on some expert opinions and papers that summarise the literature. Supervision is defined very differently across professions and across the world, and as far as possible, I have avoided using those studies that consider supervision as serving a purely educative or training function, or studies that only examine "live" supervision without a reflective component. In order to fit this chapter to the needs of today's audience, I have also limited the papers cited to those published after 1996.

The supervisory alliance

According to Webber and Deroche (2016) among others, the supervisory alliance is well established as the foundation of supervision. The supervisory alliance is the supervision equivalent of the therapeutic alliance between counsellor and client (Watkins, 2014), and so research on the online therapeutic alliance may shed light on the online supervisory alliance. Evidence suggests that a strong working alliance between counsellor and client is one of the most robust predictors of therapeutic outcome (Martin, Garske, & Davis, 2000), and recent research has found that it is possible to create strong, stable working alliances in online counselling (Andersson, et al, 2012; Knaeversrud & Maercker, 2007; Prado & Meyer, 2004).

Coker, Jones, Harbach and Staples (2002) found that counsellor trainees whose supervision was delivered through three different modalities – in-person, live text chat, and live text chat with video – perceived the supervisory alliance as being equally effective across all conditions. Studies by Reese, Aldarondo, Anderson, Lee, Miller, and Burton (2009), Rousmaniere and Frederickson (2013) and Sørlie, Gammon, Bergvik, and Sexton (1999) also detected no differences between the quality of the supervisory alliance formed in-person and that formed online.

Bussey (2015) compared the supervision experiences of ninety early-career counsellor supervisees, sixty of whom had in-person supervision and thirty of whom had video or blended video and in-person supervision. She found that across all categories, supervisees who felt that the supervisory alliance was strong were more satisfied with supervision. Notably, online supervisees were more satisfied with their supervision than their peers who were supervised in person, and rated their online supervisors more highly on factors such as warmth, friendliness, supportiveness, rapport, resourcefulness and practicality.

Unique factors in online supervision/reflection in online supervision

Speech and language therapy (SaLT) trainees having online video supervision of in-person clinical work have been very positive when asked to evaluate their supervision (Carlin, Milam, Carlin, & Owen, 2012). The majority of the supervisees polled in this study said that they believed they had at least as much supervision as their peers who were supervised in-person, and reported that online supervision was more accessible, more flexible and led to more immediate feedback.

Reindl, Engelhardt, and Zauter (2015) assert that email supervision has an advantage over in-person supervision as it gives extra space for reflection in three ways. Firstly, the act of writing encourages the supervisee to reflect upon the problems and emotions around the subject matter. Secondly, as email supervision is asynchronous, the supervisor and supervisee can also take extra time to reflect when reading or writing a response. Finally, the supervisor and supervisee can refer back to the email exchange afterwards, perhaps tracking the supervision process over time. This may be part of the reason why supervisees in other studies have reported that text-based online supervision stimulates more complex, reflective thinking which generates more insight (Fialkov, Haddad, & Gagliardi, 2001; Gammon, Sørlie, Bergvik, & Høifødt, 1998) (see also chapter one).

Recordings have long been used as a means of evaluating supervisees' work, and text-based online counselling provides us with a readymade recording of the session. The supervisor can build a clearer picture of the session by reading through the text rather than relying on the subjective recollections of the supervisee, whose recall may be incomplete or distorted by time. If the online supervision is also conducted by text, the record may be retained by the supervisee as an aide-mémoire.

Text-based supervision records can be reread repeatedly, each time focusing on a different aspect of the exchange. For example, the supervisee could first focus on the supervisor's emotional support and concrete advice on how to work with the client in the next session. On a second read-through, the supervisee could concentrate on how she presents her narrative about the client, and what this might say about their relationship and therapeutic alliance. A third read-through might reveal patterns in the interactions between supervisor and supervisee, which could potentially inform the supervisees' professional development. Reflecting on group supervision of online counsellors, Suler (2001) observes that rereading group supervision emails can not only serve as a memory refresher, but can also give insight into the group process.

Feelings of distance and presence in online supervision

Sørlie, Gammon, Bergvik, and Sexton (1999) studied six pairs of psychiatrists and trainees engaged in online supervision of in-person psychotherapy work in rural Norway. The supervision pairs alternated between in-person and videoconferencing format over ten sessions, and both supervisors and supervisees reported being better prepared and more self-disciplined in online supervision. The online supervision sessions were less likely to be interrupted by phone calls or visits, and the majority of the supervisees found that they spent more time mentally preparing for the online sessions.

Similarly, in a study of counselling trainees having online video supervision, supervisees felt that online supervision was more structured and rigid than in-person supervision, which some felt was a positive attribute (Reese, Aldarondo, Anderson, Lee, Miller, & Burton, 2009). More structured supervision sessions allowed supervisees to remain more goal-focused, which was perceived as increasing efficiency. However, when comparing the two conditions, the supervisor believed that video supervision encouraged interactions that were less personal, more intellectual, and focused more on reporting than collaborative dialogue. The supervisory alliance was rated by the supervisees as equally strong in both conditions, but online supervisees also reported feeling less intimacy with their supervisor. A supervisee participating in another study felt that the perceived lack of intimacy in online supervision created a more productive professional relationship, saying: "I think also it helped keep things very professional. We didn't sit and gossip or anything like that where maybe if I had a supervisor in person that might have happened a little more. We kept things very professional" (Carlin, Milam, Carlin, & Owen, 2012, p. 33).

Most supervisees in the Sørlie study noticed less eye contact and fewer non-verbal cues, which led to a feeling of increased distance from their supervisors in online supervision sessions. Supervisees responded to this feeling in two very different ways – some supervisees felt more able to be vulnerable and self-disclose during video sessions, while others found they intellectualised more. The authors suggested that the differences in how supervisees found online and in-person supervision sessions could be used to help the supervisees' professional development, acting as grist to the mill of the supervision process. Interacting both in-person and online enabled the supervisor to see this difference in supervisees' interpersonal interaction across modalities, which would otherwise have remained hidden.

Reese, Aldarondo, Anderson, Lee, Miller, and Burton (2009) wondered if the supervisees who prefered the distance and rigidity of video supervision were more avoidant of emotional intimacy and self-disclosure. Gammon, Sørlie, Bergvik, and Høifødt (1998) came to similar conclusions, and suggested that it is possible that the supervisees that are most drawn to online supervision are the least suitable, as the modality may facilitate the operation of problematic defence mechanisms.

Reflective questions

• What might be the advantages and disadvantages of being more mentally prepared for online supervision sessions? Is preparing more necessarily preparing "better"? What are your responses, from the points of view of both a supervisor and a supervisee?

• When you communicate with someone via text or video, do you sense their presence differently to when you communicate in-person? How might this phenomenon transfer into your online supervision?

Anxiety in working with technology

Anyone attempting to learn how to use a new computer program can testify that working with unfamiliar technology can provoke a range of emotional reactions. Both supervisors and supervisees may have emotional responses to the experience of online supervision which have the potential to affect the supervision process. Supervisors and supervisees have reported feelings of vulnerability, exposure, loss of control, discomfort, and defensiveness when working online (Gammon, Sørlie, Bergvik, & Høifødt, 1998; Graf & Stebnicki, 2002; Sørlie, Gammon, Bergvik, & Sexton, 1999).

The aforementioned study by Sørlie, Gammon, Bergvik, and Sexton (1999) found that while videoconferencing and in-person supervision sessions did not differ on the quality of the communication or the supervisory alliance, supervisees did score higher on disturbance by "external factors and/or unpleasant emotions" (p. 454). When interviewed, some supervisees reported feeling anxiety about technology at the start of the study, and these anxious feelings were linked to feeling more exposed and less in control. These feelings diminished over time but did not disappear completely over the course of the study, which involved five online supervision sessions. However, these unpleasant emotions were not found to dissuade supervisees from participating in online supervision – in fact several supervisees claimed that the study should have been extended, as it took the full five online supervision sessions to feel comfortable and competent in using the technology (Gammon, Sørlie, Bergvik, & Høifødt, 1998). The authors recommend that supervisors remain aware of the possibility of supervisees feeling anxiety over the new technology, and encourage them to reflect on it openly.

Online supervision removes some of the non-verbal cues that we follow during in-person supervision. This may increase both supervisors' and supervisees' sense of ambiguity, leaving more room for interpretation. The speed of reply in email supervision (or lack thereof) may also lead to anxieties for supervisors and supervisees, as they project their own fears and expectations onto the empty inbox

(*Why haven't they replied yet? Why have they replied so quickly? Was it something I said?*). This ambiguity can lead to the personal processes of the supervisor and supervisee becoming more central to the supervision, as the impressions of each other become shaped by projection and transference (Barak & Suler, 2008). Sørlie, Gammon, Bergvik, and Sexton (1999) say that online supervisors who have "a non-responsive analytic style" (p. 459) may compound supervisees' uncertainties. To alleviate the anxiety somewhat, Luke & Gordon (2016) recommend that supervisors pay close attention to the processes and dynamics in email supervision, attending both to the content of the messages and how the messages are communicated. Suler (2001) recommends counsellors in online peer supervision groups watch for ambiguity and seek clarification whenever in doubt about the tone or meaning of a communication. However, this approach may not be compatible with all theoretical approaches to supervision.

It is unclear whether these results indicate that online supervision is qualitatively different to in-person supervision, or if the studies highlight supervisees' discomfort at a new way of conducting supervision.

The studies mentioned here investigated supervisees' evaluation of online supervision which occurred over a low number of sessions; it is possible that feelings of distance and anxiety would have lessened over time. After twenty-five hours of supervising online, one supervisor said, "I think my perceptions of the technology changed, partly due to feeling confident about the factual characteristics and partly due to my conscious awareness of its effects on me. As I progressed towards a greater awareness and understanding of these factors [fantasies and anxiety towards the technology], I think my ability to associate freely, as well as to guide the candidates, improved" (Gammon, Sørlie, Bergvik, & Høifødt, 1998, p. 415).

Reflective questions

- What are your fantasies and anxieties about technology? Where do they come from?
- Transference can affect our relationships with people, but also our relationships with objects. Think about your computer, or the device that you use to access the internet most often. If it had a gender, what would it be? An age? A personality? How might these perceptions shape how you interact with the device and with people on the internet?
- Think of a memorable time that technology has failed you – perhaps during an online session, or when trying to access something important online. What emotions and thoughts came up for you at the time? Describe them in as much detail as possible. When else in your life have you felt that way?

Unique factors in group supervision

Online group supervision can be enormously beneficial to online counsellors, giving participants access to the knowledge and expertise of colleagues around the world.

Nelson, Nichter, and Henriksen (2010) studied two groups of counsellor trainees, one engaged in online group supervision and the other engaged in-person group supervision, and found that the groups were equally satisfied with their supervision. A study by Reese, Aldarondo, Anderson, Lee, Miller, and Burton (2009) had similar results, finding that counsellor trainees in a blended supervision group rated their satisfaction with supervision and the supervisory alliance as being equal in both in-person and video-based group supervision.

Cummings (2002) conducted a qualitative analysis of the text created during online peer group supervision with counsellor trainees. In advance of each session, one supervisee sent out an email presenting a clinical case which was then discussed in the live chat supervision group. The analysis showed that supervisees found the experience valuable, forming an honest and communicative group which noticed and used parallel process effectively. The supervisees reported increased self-disclosure and decreased inhibition, which we have also seen in online supervision for individuals (e.g., Sørlie, Gammon, Bergvik & Sexton, 1999). Other empirical studies have also found that counsellor trainees judge group email and live chat supervision to be effective (e.g., Butler & Constantine, 2006; Gainor & Constantine, 2002). Supervisees in Nelson's 2010 study rated the alliance between group members highly, with one supervisee saying, "it seemed like a really safe and almost like an intimate environment that we were able to talk freely and trust each other" (p. 10).

Suler (2001) reflects on creating and managing an email-based peer supervision group where qualified counsellors discuss clinical cases they encounter in their online counselling. Suler recommends that facilitators apply many of the same principles as they would when setting up an in-person peer supervision group – consider the number of group members, how they are selected, the skill mix and personalities involved, and set clear ground rules. The facilitators should also be aware of each group member's personal competence and attitude to online counselling and online communication more generally, as this may affect how they interact with the group. Rousmaniere, Abbass, Frederickson, Henning, and Taubner (2014) describe running an online video supervision group for licenced clinicians working psychodynamically with in-person clients, and they mention group cohesion as the biggest challenge with an online supervision group. To offset this, the authors advise that supervisors take care to get to know the individuals in the group and collaborate with supervisees to identify their learning needs. In a related piece of advice on how to maximise the benefit for all group members, Elliott, Abbass, and Cooper (2016) advise that when running groups based on a specific psychotherapeutic model, facilitators recruit group members who are similarly confident and competent with the model being used.

What do we need for good online supervision?

Supervisor qualities

Sørlie, Gammon, Bergvik, and Sexton (1999) recommend that supervisors who are uncomfortable working with technology and are unwilling to work at it do not participate in online supervision. Abbass et al (2011) assert that the supervisor can contribute to the strength of the supervisory alliance by being engaged, dedicated to the task, and comfortable with online supervision, implying that an uncomfortable supervisor will contribute to a weaker alliance. This is in line with Bernard and Goodyear's advice for supervisors to become skilled with whatever method of supervision they choose as "supervision will fall flat if the method is used poorly" (Bernard & Goodyear, 2009, p. 242). According to some online supervisors, a detached, analytical style of supervision may be less suitable for online work (Sørlie, Gammon, Bergvik, & Sexton, 1999; Suler 2001), and the ideal online supervisor would be responsive and outgoing (Gammon, Sørlie, Bergvik & Høifødt, 1998).

Reindl, Engelhardt, and Zauter (2015) found that 22.7 per cent of supervisors who responded to a survey used insecure email to communicate with online supervisees and were ill-informed about the data security issues that this raises. To provide ethical online supervision, supervisors should be competent with the technology that they use and comply with best practice in data protection and confidentiality.

Supervisee qualities

Supervisees interviewed by Gammon, Sørlie, Bergvik, and Høifødt (1998) suggested that online supervision is more suited to supervisees who are flexible, pragmatic, and secure. Conn et al (2009) conducted a study that looked at trainee counsellors receiving either in-person or blended supervision. Surveys showed that supervisees who felt more technologically competent were likely to feel more positive about online supervision, which indicates that working on reducing anxiety and increasing feelings of technological competence may be a good first step for supervisees considering working online.

Technological reliability

Although counsellor trainees engaging in blended supervision have reported being equally satisfied with online and in-person supervision, these comments often come with the caveat "if the technology is reliable" (Reese, Aldarondo, Anderson, Lee, Miller, & Burton, 2009, p. 360). Videoconferencing can be particularly prone to technological failures as it requires a lot of bandwidth. Rousmaniere (2014) advises supervision pairs to only engage in video supervision if they are aware of and comfortable with the frequent network and connectivity issues that arise with videoconferencing. He also recommends having a backup plan in case the technology fails, as do Nelson, Nichter, and Henriksen (2010). It is possible that some of the differences that we perceive between in-person and online supervision are not due to the supervision happening online per se, but due to technological issues affecting the supervision. For example, supervisees have speculated that perhaps video supervision feels more structured and less spontaneous as poor internet connectivity can often lead to you "talking over" your conversation partner, interrupting the flow of conversation (Sørlie, Gammon, Bergvik, & Sexton, 1999). Experiencing this could be embarrassing and anxiety-provoking for the supervisee, who may feel more inhibited in future conversations as she tries to prevent this from happening again.

Limitations of the research

In-person supervision research is still a relatively new field (Watkins, 2014), and online supervision is still in its infancy. Many of the limitations of in-person supervision research are transferred across to research into online supervision, such as small sample sizes and relying on self-report measures.

Studies examining online supervision of trainees engaged in in-person work can shed light on facets of the online supervision experience – the potential for building and maintaining a supervisory alliance, the efficacy and effectiveness of online vs. in-person supervision, and specific communication differences across different modalities. However, there are elements of these studies that can't be generalised to online supervision of qualified professionals engaging in online counselling, so we must be careful not to over-interpret the results. Many of the aforementioned studies recommend building a stable in-person relationship between supervisor and supervisee before transitioning to online supervision (Gammon, Sørlie, Bergvik, & Høifødt, 1998; Nelson, Nichter, & Henriksen, 2010; Sørlie, Gammon, Bergvik, & Sexton, 1999). However, this advice is likely to be less relevant to professionals working exclusively online.

Trainees may also have different supervision needs to more experienced counsellors. According to the Integrated Development Model of supervision, counsellors at the first stage of development are emotionally and intellectually focused mainly on themselves, with high insecurity, self-consciousness and high uncertainty about their work (Stoltenberg & Delworth, 1987; Stoltenberg & MacNeill, 1997). It is possible that the ambiguity of online supervision heightens these feelings, and thus online supervision may be less suitable for inexperienced counsellors. Miller, Miller, Burton, Sprang, and Adams (2003) suggest that online supervision requires supervisees to be self-directed learners with advanced competencies in some areas, and so not all trainees will be suitable for online supervision. However, online supervision can also "stretch" supervisees into growing in competencies, and one study found that supervisees felt that online supervision encouraged them to seek out internet resources, becoming more independent learners (Carlin, Milam, Carlin, & Owen, 2012).

It is probable that attitudes to and knowledge of technology have changed significantly in the past twenty years, and perhaps the findings of some of the earlier papers cited here would not be replicated if the studies were re-run today. The majority of the more recent papers on the subject (e.g., Abbass, et al, 2011; Bussey, 2015; Conn, et al, 2016; Rousmaniere & Frederickson, 2013) found that supervisees who were supervised online were at least as satisfied as those supervised in-person. Additionally, the technology used today is significantly more sophisticated, perhaps lessening the sense of distance (or increasing the sense of presence) experienced by supervisor and supervisee.

Reflective questions

- How would you determine if a supervisee was suitable for online supervision, or suitable to be an online counsellor?
- How would you assess your own suitability for online work?
- How has your attitude to technology and online work changed in the past twenty years?

Looking to the future

Some counsellors have argued against online supervision, saying, "Just because something can be done does not necessarily mean it should be done" (Greenwald, 2001, p. 12). I would argue that just because something has not been done in the past does not necessarily mean it should *not* be done. Concerns are often raised about online work – whether it is possible to create and maintain a therapeutic or supervisory alliance online, whether it is possible too for supervisees to learn effectively online, etc. – yet empirical and anecdotal evidence does not support these fears (Rousmaniere, 2014).

As mentioned earlier, we know that developments in supervision tend to follow earlier developments in counselling (Bernard & Goodyear, 2004; Clingerman & Bernard, 2004; Leddick & Bernard, 1980). If this trend is replicated in online work, we can expect an explosion of research and analysis over the next few years, helping us to build an accurate portrait of online supervision. I would expect to see more research on:

- the efficacy and effectiveness of online supervision of qualified counsellors across a range of modalities, including video, live text, email and online message boards
- research into the models of online supervision that are best suited to online work

- the qualities and competencies that are important for online supervisors and supervisees
- the supervisory alliance in online supervision of online counselling
- the applicability of theories of online communication to online supervision – is the online disinhibition effect seen in online supervision? To what degree, and does it differ across modalities? Can social information processing theory account for any of the differences between online and in-person supervision?

Online work been called the "wild west" of counselling (Rousmaniere, 2014) – a huge area which may lead to exciting new discoveries, while also containing many risks and unknowns. There are many pioneers in online supervision who are doing innovative work, but without research into the process and outcomes of online supervision, we cannot realise the full potential of these projects. Conscientious, impartial research into the advantages and disadvantages of online supervision, and the differences and similarities with in-person supervision, will help to bridge the gap between the enthusiasts and the sceptics, allowing us to build a truly evidence-based online practice.

References

Abbass, A., Arthey, S., Elliott, J., Fedak, T., Nowoweiski, D., Markovski, J., & Nowoweiski, S. (2011). Web-conference supervision for advanced psychotherapy training: A practical guide. *Psychotherapy, 48(2)* 109–118.

Andersson, G., Paxling, B., Wiwe, M., Vernmark, K., Felix, C. B., Lundborg, L., & Carlbring, P. (2012). Therapeutic alliance in guided internet-delivered cognitive behavioural treatment of depression, generalized anxiety disorder and social anxiety disorder. *Behaviour Research and Therapy, 50(9)*: 544–550.

Bambling, M., King, R., Raue, P., Schweitzer, R., & Lambert, W. (2006). Clinical supervision: Its influence on client-rated working alliance and client symptom reduction in the brief treatment of major depression. *Psychotherapy Research, 16(3)*: 317–331.

BACP (2016). *BACP Register of Counsellors & Psychotherapists: A Registrant's Guide to Supervision.* Lutterworth: BACP.

Barak, A., & Suler, J. (2008). Reflections on the psychology and social science of cyberspace. *Psychological Aspects of Cyberspace: Theory, Research, Applications*: 1–12.

Bernard, J. M., & Goodyear, R. K. (2009). *Fundamentals of Clinical Supervision (4th edn).* Boston: Pearson Education.

Bernard, J. M., & Goodyear, R. K. (2014). *Fundamentals of Clinical Supervision (5th edn).* Upper Saddle River, NJ: Pearson Education.

British Association for Behavioural & Cognitive Psychotherapies (2016). *Standards of Conduct, Performance and Ethics.* Bury BABCP.

British Psychoanalytic Council (2011). *Code of Ethics.*

British Psychological Society (2009). *Code of Ethics and Conduct: Guidance Published by the Ethics Committee of the British Psychological Society.* Leicester: BPS.

Bussey, L. E. (2015). *The Supervisory Relationship: How Style and Working Alliance Relate to Satisfaction among Cyber and Face-to-Face Supervisees.* PhD diss., University of Tennessee. Available online at: http://trace.tennessee.edu/utk_graddiss/3564.

Butler, S., & Constantine, M. (2006). Web-based peer supervision, collective self-esteem, and case conceptualization ability in school counselor trainees. *Professional School Counseling, 10(2)*: 146–152.

Callahan, J. L., Almstrom, C. M., Swift, J. K., Borja, S. E., & Heath, C. J. (2009). Exploring the contribution of supervisors to intervention outcomes. *Training and Education in Professional Psychology, 3(2)*: 72–77.

Carlin, C. H., Milam, J. L., Carlin, E. L., & Owen, A. (2012). Promising practices in e-supervision: Exploring graduate speech-language pathology interns' perceptions. *International Journal of Telerehabilitation, 4(2)*: 25–38.

Clingerman, T. L. & Bernard, J. M. (2004). An investigation of the use of e-mail as a supplemental modality for clinical supervision. *Counselor Education and Supervision, 44(2)*: 82–95.

Coker, J. K., Jones, W. P., Harbach, R. L., & Staples, P. (2002). Cyber-supervision in the first practicum: Implications for research and practice. *Guidance and Counselling, 18(1)*: 33–38.

Conn, S. R., Roberts, R. L., Powell, B. M., Journal, S., April, N., Conn, S. R., & Powell, B. M. (2016). Attitudes and satisfaction with a hybrid model of counseling supervision. *International Forum of Educational Technology & Society, 12(2)*: 298–306.

Cummings, P. (2002). Cybervision: Virtual peer group counselling supervision: Hindrance or help? *Counselling and Psychotherapy Research, 2(4)*: 223–229.

Elliott, J., Abbass, A., & Cooper, J. (2016). International group supervision using videoconference technology. In: T. Rousmaniere & E. Renfro-Michel, *Using Technology to Enhance Clinical Supervision*. Alexandria, VA: American Counselling Association, pp. 191–202.

Fialkov, C. Haddad, D., & Gagliardi, J. (2001). Face to face on the line: An invitation to learn from online supervision. *AAMFT Supervision Bulletin, Summer*: 1–3.

Gainor, K. A., & Constantine, M. G. (2002). Multicultural group supervision: A comparison of inperson versus web-based formats. *Professional School Counseling, 6(2)*: 104–111.

Gammon, D., Sørlie, T., Bergvik, S., & Høifødt, T. S. (1998). Psychotherapy supervision conducted by videoconferencing: a qualitative study of users' experiences. *Journal of Telemedicine and Telecare, 4 Suppl 1* (December 2015): 33–35.

Gay, P. (1998). *Freud: A life for Our Time*. New York: Norton.

Gilbert, M., & Evans, K. (2000). *Psychotherapy Supervision*. Buckingham: Open University Press.

Graf, N. M., & Stebnicki, M. A. (2002). Using E-mail for clinical supervision in practicum: A qualitative analysis. *Journal of Rehabilitation, 68(3)*: 41–49.

Goodyear, R. K., & Bernard, J. M. (1998). Clinical supervision: Lessons from the literature. *Counselor Education & Supervision, 38*: 6–22.

Greenwald, B. C. (2001). Cybersupervision: Some ethical issues. *AAMFT Supervision Bulletin, Summer*: 1–3.

Jencius, M., Baltimore, M. L., & Getz, H. G. (2010). Innovative uses of technology in clinical supervision. *State of the art in clinical supervision*: 63–85.

Jones, G., & Stokes, A. (2009). *Online Counselling: A Handbook for Practitioners*. Basingstoke: Palgrave Macmillan.

Knaevelsrud, C., & Maercker, A. (2007). Internet-based treatment for PTSD reduces distress and facilitates the development of a strong therapeutic alliance: A randomized controlled clinical trial. *BMC Psychiatry, 7(1)*: 13.

Ladany, N., & Inman, A. G. (2012). Training and supervision. *Oxford Handbook of Counseling Psychology*: 179–207.

Leddick, G. R., & Bernard, J. M. (1980). The history of supervision: A critical review. *Counselor Education and Supervision, 19(3)*: 186–196.

Luke, M. & Gordon, C. (2016). Clinical Supervision via E-Mail: A Review of the Literature and Suggestions for Practice. In: T. Rousmaniere & E. Renfro-Michel, *Using Technology to Enhance Clinical Supervision* (pp. 117–134). Alexandria, VA: American Counselling Association.

Martin, D., Garske, J., & Davis, M. (2000) Relation of the therapeutic alliance with other outcome and other variables: A meta-analytic review. *Journal of Consulting and Clinical Psychology, 68:* 438–450.

Miller, T. W., Miller, J. M., Burton, D., Sprang, R., & Adams, J. (2003). Telehealth: A model for clinical supervision in allied health. *Internet Journal of Allied Health Sciences and Practice, 1(2)*: 1–11.

Nelson, J. A., Nichter, M., & Henriksen, R. (2010). On-line supervision and face-to-face supervision in the counseling internship An exploratory study of similarities and differences. *Vistas 2010.* Available online at: www.counselingoutfitters.com/vistas/vistas10/Article_46.pdf.

Pilling, S., & Roth, A. D. (2014). The competent clinical supervisor. *The Wiley International Handbook of Clinical Supervision* 20–37.

Prado, S., & Meyer, S. B. (2004). *Evaluation of the Working Alliance of an Asynchronous Therapy Via the Internet.* MA dissertation. Sao Paulo: University of Sao Paulo.

Reese, R. J., Aldarondo, F., Anderson, C. R., Lee, S.-J., Miller, T. W., & Burton, D. (2009). Telehealth in clinical supervision: A comparison of supervision formats. *Journal of Telemedicine and Telecare, 15*: 356–361.

Reindl, R. (2015). Psychosoziale Onlineberatung – von der praktischen zur geprüften Qualität. *E-beratungsjournal, 11(1)*: 55–68.

Reindl, R., Engelhardt, E., & Zauter, S. (2015). *Abschlussbericht: Online-Supervision–Systematische Bestandsaufnahme eines neuen Arbeitsfeldes.* Available online at: www.e-beratungsinstitut.de/wordpress/wp-content/uploads/2016/03/Abschlussbericht-Projekt-Online-Supervision.pdf.

Rousmaniere, T. (2014). Using technology to enhance clinical supervision and training. *The Wiley International Handbook of Clinical Supervision*: 204–237.

Rousmaniere, T., Abbass, A., Frederickson, J., Henning, I., & Taubner, S. (2014). Videoconference for psychotherapy training and supervision: Two case examples. *American Journal of Psychotherapy, 68(2)*: 231–50.

Rousmaniere, T., & Frederickson, J. (2013). Internet-based one-way-mirror supervision for advanced psychotherapy training. *Clinical Supervisor, 32(1)*: 40–55.

Sorlie, T., Gammon, D., Bergvik, S., & Sexton, H. (1999). Psychotherapy supervision face-to-face and by video conferencing: A comparative study. *British Journal of Psychotherapy, 15(4)*: 452–462.

Stoltenberg, C. D., & Delworth, U. (1987). *Supervising Counselors and Therapists: A Developmental Approach.* San Francisco: Jossey-Bass.

Stoltenberg, C. D. & McNeill, B. W. (1997). Clinical supervision from a developmental perspective: Research and practice. *Handbook of psychotherapy supervision*: 184–202.

Suler, J. R. (2001). The online clinical case study group: An e-mail model. *Cyberpsychology & Behavior, 4(6)*: 711–722.

UK Council for Psychotherapy (2012). *Supervision Policy.* London: UKCP.

Watkins, C. E., & Ph, D. (2014). The supervisory alliance: A half century of theory, practice, and research in critical perspective. *American Journal of Psychotherapy, 68(1)*: 19–55.

Webber, J. M., & Deroche, M. D. (2016). Technology and accessibility in clinical supervision: Challenges and solutions. In: T. Rousmaniere & E. Renfro-Michel, *Using Technology to Enhance Clinical Supervision* (pp. 67–86). Alexandria, VA: American Counselling Association.

Wetchler, J., Trepper, T., McCollum, E., & Nelson, T. S. (1993). Videotape supervision via long-distance telephone. *The American Journal of Family Therapy, 21*: 242–247.

Chapter 3

Meandering through models: can face-to-face supervision models be used for online supervision?

Anne Stokes

In response to the question in the chapter title, it would be easy simply to say, "Yes, if you think it through" and leave it at that! However, that doesn't answer the underlying enquiry, which is more about "how" and about issues, rather than a simple demand. In a short chapter, it is impossible to look at the multitude of f2f supervision models and their compatibility with online supervision, so I have chosen to look at just a few of the most well-known. In general terms, I would expect most models to be able to be used online if one looks at the underlying principles. What I think is necessary in applying them is to consider if there are any aspects that couldn't transfer to online working, and importantly, what might be the extra considerations or expansions of aspects of the original model.

Remember that these are solely my interpretations or adaptions of the models and that therefore the originators, and/or you, might well use the same base f2f model but come up with completely different ideas about using it in online supervision and produce a completely different set of adaptations. I rarely accept that there is only one way of doing something. In considering these models, they have of necessity been simply and very briefly outlined. To do each one justice demands a complete book. I have listed the works on which I have based my explorations in the reference section at the end.

Perhaps the best-known supervision model is that of Proctor and Inskipp (Proctor, 2000), who use the following terms to describe the 3 main foci in supervising f2f counselling:

- Formative
- Restorative
- Normative

The formative process in supervision is about developing skills, understanding and abilities of the supervisee. In f2f work, this would be done through exploring and reflecting on the supervisee's work with clients. This is equally so in online supervision, but there would be an extra dimension: that of developing skills and abilities with regard to the particular medium. Both technological issues and issues which may arise specifically with online clients, such as disinhibition, would fall into this category.

The "normative" aspect provides a check on the quality of the work with client, highlighted in *BACP's Ethical Framework* (Bond, 2016). Again, there are similar aspects in online supervision to those present in f2f work, including consideration of the principles for ethical working, organisational and professional requirements – in other words, does the work conform to widely held norms within the therapeutic community? However, in addition in online supervision, it would be also necessary to consider the supplementary guidance given for example by BACP for working online (Bond, 2015) or by the Association of Counsellors and Therapists Online (ACTO, www.acto-org.uk).

The "restorative" function responds to supervisees who may have been affected by their clients' issues or trauma. Online supervisees are no less affected in this way than f2f, and these will be worked with in the supervision sessions. There may be other areas of restoration not experienced in f2f work. For example, clients who "disappear" occurs more often online; it is perhaps even more stressful working online with a young client or one who becomes suicidal. Isolation, sitting too long at a computer and dealing with the IT gremlins are all areas which can benefit from the restorative nature of good online supervision.

Consideration of the Proctor and Inskipp model demonstrates immediately the reason I say above that it is possible to adapt many f2f models, if one considers the extra online dimension.

Another well-known f2f model is the cyclical model (Page & Woskett, 2000). It was a key part of my own integrative model of f2f supervision, so it was important for me to see if I could also use it in my online supervision.

Sometimes when I consider a f2f model, it is hard to work out how, or indeed, if, it might work online. So below, in the session outline, I attempt to show how this model might work – very briefly. This is not *"the truth"* – simply my version of how it might happen in one session. In case you are not familiar with the model, I will first give a very short overview. I have chosen to look at the model in a synchronous setting – this could be voice or video. In my experience, this model most readily adapts to live online supervision. When reflecting on my email supervision with supervisees, while I am aware that I do use this model, it perhaps is a less 'smooth' adaptation. I am able to note all the stages and sub-divisions over a series of exchanges, but rarely within one single email exchange.

The model

There are 5 stages and each stage has five sub-divisions. It is an attempt to give a framework to the supervision process – it is a map, and should be seen as flexible rather than as a rigid structure.

1. Contract: this is the overall agreement for supervision *per se*, but also the agreement for that session. Its five divisions encompass ground rules, boundaries, accountability, expectations, and relationship.

2. Focus: this is both the point of entry into the "work" and also the material under consideration at any particular moment – the locus of attention. The sub-divisions here are: issue, objectives, presentation, approach, priorities.
3. Space: sometimes termed "creative play space", this is where the heart of the supervision takes place. It's about exploration, experimentation, reflection, insight and understanding. Its five sub-divisions are: collaboration, investigation, challenge, containment, affirmation. Online supervisors need to think about (and practice) ways that they can encourage creativity in this medium.
4. Bridge: this is what it sounds like – the bridge back from the supervision process to the counsellor's work. Here consolidation, information giving, goal setting, action taking, and client's perspective are the five sub divisions.
5. Review: this last stage is both a continuous process, and also involves periodic more major review of the process of supervision. Routinely, in each supervision session, there is a review of what has been achieved and what needs to be carried forward. So, the subdivisions here are: feedback, grounding, evaluation, assessment, re-contracting.

Crucially, within a supervision session not all sub-divisions may be present each time.

So, let's consider an online supervision session.

1. Adele has come to an online synchronous text supervision session with Lisa, and in the first few minutes of the session they *contract* for that session. Adele states that today she would like to bring two clients and asks Lisa to be the one to watch how time is allocated during the session to leave her free to think about her clients (ground rules/expectations). She also tells Lisa that she has signed up for a course on SFBT in an Online Context, as in the last session they had discussed the fact that she was beginning to take short term agency clients without having any training to work this way online (boundaries/accountability). Lisa asks whether there was anything they needed to come back to from that session as when she had looked back over the transcript, she had wondered if she had appeared rather authoritarian at one point (relationship).

2. To *focus,* Adele presents her first online client, outlining the *issues* as she sees them, and says that she wants to have a clearer sense of how her client relates to people *(objective and possibly priority)*. She says how they have been working together (approach) and recognises that the *priority* is about how she and the client relate, which is somehow different from her f2f clients. She states that she is aware that she and her client are exploring f2f relationships, yet they have an online relationship, so how does that affect the process?

3. In the *space,* Lisa asks Adele if she has an image of the relationship. She comes up with a metaphor which they expand and explore together (collaboration and investigation) using an online whiteboard. Lisa facilitates Adele as she works with anger she feels towards her client and way she appears to use people (containment), and notices that anger has been a theme with several clients recently

(challenge), and affirms Adele's awareness that this is something she may need to explore further in her own therapy as well as here in supervision.

4. Adele then thinks about the insights into her relationship with this client (consolidation) and Lisa asks if she knows about an article about online relationships which might also be useful (information giving). Adele decides that she does not want to set any goals or plan any action with this client (bridge). Lisa asks if she has any sense of what the client might say if she heard Adele decide that no action was needed. Adele is comfortable that she would agree! (client perspective).

2. They return to *focusing* on the second client, with Adele outlining the priority as being how to address the client's difficulties in regularly attending online sessions. She tells Lisa what she has done already in this area (approach).

3. In the *space*, Adele decides to "become" the client and asks Lisa to be her (the online therapist) addressing the issue with the client. Adele experiences huge ambivalence towards Lisa as the online counsellor, and they explore what might be happening both in the "here and now" and also in the "there and then".

4. This has helped Adele to have a greater understanding of what might be going on for her client (client perspective) and some sense of how she might take this forward (goals and action).

5. As they come towards the end of the session, they *review* and Lisa *feeds back* to Adele that she has noticed how she is gaining confidence in experimenting in her online supervision sessions, and Adele agrees that she now feels safe enough in the relationship to risk trying things out. They are both quiet, not typing for a few moments and each reflect on the session (grounding) and then, as they always do, they look at what has been useful and what they might have done differently in the session (evaluation). Adele tells Lisa that as part of her appraisal in an online agency where she works part-time, there has been a suggestion that supervisors should be asked to give a report (assessment) and asks if they could spend some time in the next session discussing this, when she will know more details (re-contracting). They check the details of the next session before ending.

What didn't happen in this imagined online session was a break down in technology! This is of course a huge difference from f2f supervision and how to deal with it must be included in the initial contract. Overall in my experience, it has been useful to have this model as part of my toolkit of online supervision and also to share it with my supervisees so that we both take some responsibility for how the process unfolds.

A brief approach to online supervision

Following on from Adele's indication in the scenario above that she was considering working briefly with online clients, it seems appropriate to consider brief online supervision approaches. In my experience, this approach to supervision works well, whether or not the supervisee works briefly with online clients because "brief interventions" is genuinely an approach, rather than a model. It is extremely collaborative. One criticism of online supervision concerns whether an hour of synchronous text work is equivalent to a similar time f2f. While I am not discussing this here, I would say that a "brief" focus helps to make effective use of the time available, both synchronously and asynchronously.

One of the basic tenets of brief work is respectful curiosity concerning the supervisee and the process of therapy. It aims to validate competence and resources, and to work to defined goals. The latter might be set each session: "What are you hoping to achieve from this session?" (or exchange of emails) It could be a longer-term goal over a number of supervision sessions: "I want to increase my ability to challenge appropriately online." The supervisor checks frequently whether and how the goals are being achieved.

Many "ways of being and working" from SFBT are useful here (e.g., looking for exceptions to problems arising in the supervisee's work or identifying pre-existing solutions). "So how have you worked with online disinhibition before? And what was helpful in the way you did that?" Generally, the focus is more on how the supervisee is working than on the client's story.

Between online supervision sessions, a helpful brief technique of ensuring that the supervisor retains an overall sense of the supervisee's work is for every client to be named in a password protected document at a set interval such as once every two months. They are then rated on a scale of zero to ten (ten being that everything is going as well as it possibly could). The supervisee writes briefly about what would be different if the next session moved up a point, and how they would recognise this. The document is attached to an encrypted email and then to the supervisor. This enables both parties to recognise if there is a need to do or be something different, or do/be more of the same.

Many online supervisors already integrate brief "techniques" into their supervision. For my part, from time to time, I find it useful to go back and see if I could do more to improve my online supervision. However, one of the criticisms of using a brief approach in online supervision is that the supervisor can come over as being very abrupt and challenging. This is particularly commented on in text based work, since there are no verbal or visual clues to "soften" the words. Therefore, in working briefly by text it is vital to maintain the "respectful curiosity" and collaborative working alliance, and to check out frequently how you are being perceived.

The process model

Peter Hawkins and Robin Shohet (2000) developed a process model as a way of looking at f2f supervision in the helping professions, which has evolved over time. They assert that differences arise in the way people are supervised due to the constant choices that supervisors encourage about what to focus on in a supervision session, rather than from developmental stages, primary tasks, or intervention styles seen in some other models.

Summing it up very briefly and possibly rather simplistically, it consists of seven possibilities, or "eyes", where the supervision process might focus. They are:

1. Reflection on the content of the counselling session. The focus is on the client.
2. Exploration of techniques and strategies used by the counsellor.
3. Exploration of the relationship.
4. The feelings of the counsellor towards the client (the counsellor's counter-transference).
5. Focus on what is happening here and now between supervisor/ supervisee as a parallel of the "there and then".
6. A focus on what is happening here and now for the supervisor (the supervisor's counter-transference).
7. Reflection on organisational/systemic issues (the context of client and the supervision) (Based on Hawkins & Shohet, 2000).

If we consider each of these "eyes" in turn, it is possible to see how the model adapts to working online, and to see some of the possible difficulties. When the supervisee "tells the story" of the session, if the session is synchronous text based, the speed of typing may mean that the session never moves beyond this stage. There are at least two ways around this: the supervisee types up the story before the session, so that it can be cut and pasted very quickly on to the screen, or an email containing the story of the session is sent to the supervisor before the session. If the supervision is by email that would happen anyway, although it would be important that this part of the email is not so long, that the supervisor must wade through pages of words.

The exploration of techniques and strategies is the same as in f2f, with the additional focus on exploring how they may have to be adapted for online work. So, for example, a supervisee may want to think about how challenges can be made online in a way which comes over to the client as supportive rather than confrontational. While this might seem to apply solely to text based work, in fact, given that only a part of the counsellor is seen in video work, they may still need to consider how their techniques and strategies are truly perceived by an online client. What might be the indications that all is not working effectively?

The exploration of the relationship is something to which most of us are used to doing in f2f supervision, and again it is solely a matter of adapting this to online work. So, the supervisor may need to "be more curious" as they are not picking up verbal clues (not even completely in video work) about how the supervisee "knows" this or that about the relationship. One of the values of working with a supervisee who uses text-based online therapy with clients is that they can send the supervisor a verbatim account to read, so the supervisor may be able to read "between the lines". Of course, if it is being sent, it must be with the client's permission, and in an encrypted document.

With the following three "eyes" parallels, transference, countertransference and projection may be experienced online (though some therapists and supervisors will recognise these phenomena using different terms). It is amazing when newly working online to discover that they can really happen, even when two people are not in the same place, or indeed, sometimes not even in the same time period! However, one of the considerations is that occasionally there could be some difficulty in terms of "eye five" in being sure that the "here and now" tells us anything about the "there and then". I am thinking about a therapist working with a f2f client but bringing them to online supervision, or even a therapist working by email with a client but receiving video supervision. There is a possibility that the difference in the medium used distorts the process.

When considering the last "eye", as well as the systemic and organisation issues which would normally be considered, there are others which are specific to online working. These could relate to the geographic contexts of any of the three parties involved (client, therapists, and supervisor), so for example, legal issues particularly with regard to online work, but also the law itself in a particular jurisdiction, consideration of support systems in a different country and so on. IT systems and security will definitely be a supervision issue from time to time; the possibility of clients falsifying their identity; and working with young people online. These are examples of issues which arise in online supervision. While the use of social media and online presence is becoming an issue for consideration by all therapists, regardless of whether they work online or not, it is likely to be a more constantly present systemic issue in online supervision.

Developmental models of supervision

There is value in considering developmental models of supervision in the context of online supervision. In f2f contexts, these developed largely in the USA from the mid-sixties onwards. Perhaps the best known of the model was fashioned by Stoltenberg and Delworth (1987). The hypothesis behind developmental models is that the supervisor needs to be able to employ a range of styles and appreciate a range of approaches. These are then used and modified with regard to the therapist's level of experience and development.

Integrating an awareness of developmental levels into online supervision seems to me to be fundamental. A supervisee may have been working as a therapist for many years and therefore may be thought of as developmentally at a high level. However, when an experienced therapist begins to work online, there may well be a regression to being a "beginner" therapist both in terms of specific skills and also in self-confidence. Thus, an online supervisor would do well to bear the developmental levels of their supervisees in mind, both as a therapist per se and an online practitioner in particular.

Level 1   Self-centred. Can I make it this work? So, the online supervisee is very concerned with the "strangeness" of working this way and whether or not they can, or even want to, do so.

Level 2   Client-centred. Can I help this online client? Am I good enough? And also occasionally, like an adolescent, being over confident and liable to rush into situations that they are not yet ready for.

Level 3   Process-centred. Concentration on how the online relationship and process is working. Able to work much more independently and confidently.

Level 4   Process-in-context-centred. The supervisee is much more interested in the online process itself. They may well be interested in the online supervision process and whether they might think about training as an online supervisor.

This ties in well with Howell's (1982) theory of competence, whereby people move for unconscious incompetence through to unconscious competence. The levels of competence tie in well with Stoltenberg and Delworth's developmental levels. As previously stated, even an experienced f2f therapist can experience these levels of competence as they begin to work online. It takes a skilful online supervisor to be able to gently challenge the supervisee to recognise that they may be unconsciously incompetent without destroying their confidence and enthusiasm for working online. Of course, there is also a danger in supervising the therapist at the unconscious competence level as they may not be keeping abreast of new developments in the online field.

Level 1   Unconscious incompetence – not knowing what you don't know.

Level 2   Conscious incompetence – being very aware of what you don't know.

Level 3   Conscious competence – knowing what to do and being able to do it, but it not being fully integrated.

Level 4   Unconscious competence – being able to work intuitively to a large extent.

As a reader, you may (or may not!) be interested to know which model I use when supervising online. As in my original f2f supervision work, I find that I do not use any one model and reject the rest. My spine is the Proctor and Inskipp model as those three elements chime with my humanistic approach to both counselling and supervision. So, in the moment, I will probably be using a mixture of these.

In terms of how I structure the synchronous session, loosely I have at the back of my mind the cyclical model of Page and Wosket. I find that this enables the session to be purposeful and effective. I do not consciously use the process model within synchronous sessions or email exchanges, but rather as a reflective tool afterwards. I will note which "eyes" we seem to use most and wonder about that, particularly in my online supervision of supervision. If I notice that we are avoiding one, or perhaps favouring another at the cost of the rest, I might consciously work to include that in sessions. It may be to do with something going on in me, or it may be something which a particular supervisee is drawing us towards or away from. Often it is useful to include the "eyes" in our periodic reviews, so that we share both a sense of what is going on and hold a joint responsibility for the online supervision process.

Developmentally, in terms of who I am working with, where supervisees are in their online journey and experience will definitely play a part.

In reading the above paragraph, you might be saying to yourself, "So what is different, then, about online supervision, and if I am a f2f supervisor, why can't I just switch to offering online supervision without all this fuss about training?" The answer in my opinion, is that while these and other models are able to be adapted very usefully to online supervision, you must be aware of how they can work online, and what are the "extras" that you need to take in to account which are specific to online work from both a therapeutic and a supervision perspective. I think it is very difficult to fully understand these without some further training. It is rather like putting together a piece of flat pack furniture. I can read the instructions and think I understand them. The actual practice may show me that I haven't! Or worse still, I may think I have succeeded, but every joiner would notice how badly I had constructed it.

So where have my meanderings taken me? They have reminded me of the value in staying open to considering existing models, of weighing them up and taking from them aspects that may inform or improve my own online supervision practice. Having explored f2f models and their suitability for online work in this chapter, I would like to highlight a question which I am sometimes asked – should f2f approaches be adapted for online work, or should new ones, specific to the medium, be developed instead. My answer is "yes"! In other words, it is not "either/or", but "and/and". If I am comfortable using a particular approach f2f, what is wrong with using it online, with thought, ethical reflection and any necessary adaptations? However, I would also suggest that few of us use "pure" models anyway, in counselling or in supervision, whether f2f or online. So, consciously or unconsciously, we probably have developed our own "new" model. In the chapter which follows, some online supervisors will discuss their own developed and developing models.

Reflective questions

- If you are a f2f supervisor, outline your model of supervision and consider whether it would adapt to online work. If so, how would you do this?
- If you are an online supervisor, reflect on how your online supervision model has evolved. In reviewing it, are there any areas you want to strengthen or any adaptations you would like to make in light of your experience of working online?
- If you are not a supervisor, think about your work with your supervisor. Has she or he shared the model of supervision that she or he uses? If so, think about how that adapts (or doesn't) to online work. If not, can you articulate a model that might be being used? You might like to share that with your supervisor!

38

References

Bond, T. (2015). *Good Practice in Action 047: Ethical Framework for the Counselling Professions Supplementary Guidance: Working Online.* Lutterworth: BACP.

Bond, T. (2016). *Ethical Framework for the Counselling Professions.* Lutterworth: BACP.

Hawkins, P. & Shohet, R. (2000). *Supervision in the Helping Professions (2nd edn).* Maidenhead: Open University Press.

Howell, W. S. (1982). *The Empathic Communicator.* Boston: Wadsworth.

Page, S. & Wosket, V. (2001). *Supervising the Counsellor: A Cyclical Model (2nd edn).* London: Routledge.

Proctor, B. (2000). *Group Supervision: A Guide to Creative Practice.* London: Sage.

Stoltenberg, C. D. & Delworth, U. (1987). *Supervising Counsellors and Therapists.* San Francisco: Jossey-Bass.

Chapter 4

New models of online supervision – (1) CLEAR

Maria O'Brien

Hello, my name is Maria O'Brien. Welcome to my contribution on how a supervision model originally designed for f2f practice can be utilised for online supervision.

Historically, the practice of supervision was overtly seen as an apprentice learning and benefiting from the experience, skills and wisdom of a "master" practitioner within the field. Whilst this practice offered a means of safeguarding clients and ensuring ethical practice, it relied on the supervisor's counselling skills being transferable into what is now seen as a different discipline and therefore one that requires specific training.

Fast forward a number of years and the results of research and development within this field have yielded various categories of supervision, recognised supervision training, and an abundance of models for traditional face-to-face practice. These developments were paralleled by advances in technology; the one telephone per household usually located in a draughty hallway was being replaced by mobile phones and computers. Over the years practitioners continued to research and explore how being technologically connected could facilitate the establishment and maintenance of therapeutic contact both practically and ethically. In partnership with professional counselling organisations, their contributions continued to provide us with an up to date set of professional standards. These BACP standards and guidelines (Anthony & Goss, 2009; Bond, 2015; Stokes 2016) can be found in the reference section at the end of the chapter and include:

* Guidelines for online counselling and supervision
* Guidelines for telephone and e-counselling competences
* And competences for training the next generation of online practitioners

Sadly, advances in the development of supervision models specifically for online practice hasn't kept pace. As a result, supervisors have become proficient in adopting face-to-face models to suit technology and their chosen medium of facilitation, such as instant messaging video conferencing or emails. From my perspective, it would seem that some models lend themselves to this process a little more easily than others, but before we delve into identifying which are more pliable, let's take a look at some of the factors for consideration before adopting a framework to be used in practice.

- How do I define supervision?
- How does this specific model fit with my beliefs about human beings and in turn my counselling approach?
- Does this model fulfil the requirements I have for my personal development either as a supervisor or supervisee?
- Is this model compatible with technology and the various mediums used to facilitate and support online supervision?
- Is this model easy to remember?

The first question focuses on a definition of supervision. I tend to favour the Hawkins & Shohet (2012) definition which states:

> Supervision is a joint endeavour in which a practitioner with the help of a supervisor, attends to their clients, themselves as part of their client practitioner relationships and the wider systemic context, and by so doing improves the quality of their work, transforms their client relationships, continuously develops themselves, their practice and the wider professions. (p. 5)

For me this definition focuses on the developmental and relational encounters therapists have with themselves, their clients and the wider system.

The second two factors take into consideration one's personal model of counselling and future development of the working triad of client, counsellor, and supervisor. As an integrative practitioner whose core counselling orientation is person centred, my model of online supervision practice is integrated via the therapeutic relationship. Lapworth, Sills, and Fish (2006) state that, "the therapeutic relationship is an essential facet of [a] multidimensional integrative framework" (p. 99). So, whilst frameworks will inform my understanding of the supervisory process, my approach and facilitation of them will be through a relational style. Hence there is congruence between my models of counselling and supervision.

The latter, an elementary but nonetheless an important question, reflects on the model's ability to provide a navigational compass for the supervision session. Once those questions have been explored and satisfactorily addressed for the individual practitioner, a final consideration is how will all of that adapt to work online. My own responses to those queries influenced my selection of the CLEAR model for practice. Developed by Peter Hawkins in the 1980s, the letters are an acronym:

- Contract
- Listen
- Explore
- Action
- Review

They offer a blend of the process and practicalities associated with supervision that invites and encourages collaboration. Despite linear listing, the model functions cyclically and oscillatory so both supervisor and supervisee can be in all the spaces at once e.g. listening to, exploring and reviewing a possible action which may lead to re-contracting the focus of the session.

Gilbert & Evans (2000) define contracting as "an agreement between the supervisor and supervisee about the goal(s) of supervision (p. 68) They go onto suggest that in the contract, the two participants focus on an agreed outcome for the supervision, which then gives a shape to the particular supervision session and defines the task for the supervisor. Hawkins and Shohet (2012) concur and suggest that, "the contracting phase of the CLEAR model starts with the end in mind and agreeing how you are going to get there" (p. 67). In my opinion this initial focus on agreeing a contract for time and focus of the session sets a tone of joint responsibility and promotes a sense of equality which challenges the concept of what Folett (1924) described as "power over" to be replaced with a sense of "power with".

Once a contract has been established there is movement towards creating an active listening space where the supervisor and supervisee can get a more detailed understanding of the issues the supervisee wishes to look at. As the process is facilitated online, supervisors and supervisees who work synchronously and asynchronously via text will have sharpened awareness of hearing via their cognitive, emotional, behavioural, and somatic responses. Drawing on these sensory cues as guidance for reflexive questioning enables both parties to examine the overt and covert impact the client is having on the supervisee and how that may influence choice of intervention.

In supervision, like therapy, it is necessary to create a safe enough space where a number of facets can be managed. These include aspects seen and unseen, conscious and unconscious processes, and material presented and then represented. The invitation for supervisee reflection on these facets offers potential for greater insight about the client, self and the therapeutic relationship, and action a process of transformational learning. Carroll (2008, p. 3) suggests that transformational learning:

> [...] enables individuals to shift gear into another way of perceiving. Part of the process in transformational learning is the evaluation of old mind sets and mental maps. With transformational learning comes new ways of perceiving and looking at situations. inking is more systemic and allows individuals to connect more to the bigger picture.

Clark (1993), in Cooper suggests:

> Transformational learning is defined as learning that induces more far-reaching change in the learner than other kinds of learning, especially learning experiences which shape the learner and produce a significant impact, or paradigm shift, which affects the learner's subsequent experiences.

In his paper on transformational learning, Taylor (1998) suggests that constructing and creating both the environment and the process of transformational learning is the responsibility of both parties. In a similar theme, Daloz (1999) used the metaphor of transformation as a journey in which the mentor or instructor served as a gatekeeper. These views appear to propose that transformational learning is rooted in an overseen collaborative environment which I believe is akin to the stages of the CLEAR model that inform practice as follow.

Contract: agreeing on the focus of session

As practitioners, contracts are central to our work. They provide containment for both parties and, if adhered to, safeguard ethical practice. As well as the overall working contract which for online supervision addresses issues relating to storage of online data, arrangements for breakdowns in technology and the use of social media, the sessional contracting/agenda within this model shapes the session.

Listen: helping the supervisee to gain insight into the situation

This aspect refers to the creation of an active listening space built on empathy and respect where the supervisee sets out the issues they wish to bring to supervision. The supervisor, via catalytic interventions, communicates they have heard and understood the issues to be explored. As this book focuses on working online, sometimes without visual and aural cues, sound is usually interpreted through the tone of text which requires regular checking of understanding. As a user of this model, I also relate this listening to the supervisor's ability to tune into and listen to themselves and their responses to the supervisee, client and any organisational issues presented.

Explore: helping the supervisee to identify patterns and themes within the therapeutic relationship and increase their awareness of the impact the situation is having on themselves

Through the use of skilled questioning and reflecting, both parties examine the impact that client material is having on all of the supervisee, paying close attention to how patterns and themes within the client's story might be informing parallel processes in the therapeutic relationship.

Working online adds another dimension in that the exploration may also focus on practicalities for example how clients cope with technology, are they on time for synchronous sessions, are there issues with internet connections? Examining these aspects in unison helps the supervisee think through possibilities for future action within therapy sessions.

Action: supporting the supervisee in committing to a way ahead and creating the next step

The insight generated can reveal options for addressing the issue the supervisee raised. This can range from continuing to work on developing the therapeutic relationship to the extreme of having to report on a safeguarding or legislative issue, which involves breaking confidentiality. In either case, the supervisor will encourage the supervisee to reflect on, develop and commit to a plan of action and how that will be carried out.

At this point I would like to stress that an action plan may range from thoughts conducting more research on a specific issue a client has brought, to involving a third party in what is deemed to be a safeguarding issue.

Review: reflecting on what has been achieved within the session, acknowledging commitments made for planned action and future review of the trialled action

I see this aspect of the model having a definite split between reviewing the supervision session – that is looking at what the supervisees will take away and how that will be fed back into practice – and reviewing (possibly at the beginning of the next session) how the action was executed and what was learned.

I see the latter three words, "what was learned", to be of great importance from both a developmental and relational perspective. Working with this model is likely to harness and increase the supervisees' skills of presentation, communication and their ability to view, re-view and perhaps reach a different balance of understanding of the issues raised.

However, as the saying goes, nothing is perfect and that is true of this model. For me, its shortcomings are rooted in the unseen, specifically the lack of overt consideration of how the culture and spiritual values of both supervisee and supervisor are likely to inform interventions. As practitioners, I hope our awareness of such issues means we invite open discussion of these and other issues with our supervisees so in turn they can extend a similar invitation to their clients.

Finally, I would like to thank you for witnessing my train of thought on how historic and recent developments in the therapeutic and technological arena have influenced the birth and continued evolvement of online counselling and supervision. Personally, this journey has crystallised the value of engaging in a supervisory process where the primary aim is learning that is transformational. I hope I have shown how the CLEAR model can provide a framework for that and that some of what has been written is informative.

References

Anthony, K. & Goss, S. (2009). *Guidelines for Online Counselling and Psychotherapy (3rd Edition), including Guidelines for Online Supervision.* Lutterworth: BACP.

Bond, T. (2015). *Good Practice in Action 047: Ethical Framework for the Counselling Professions Supplementary Guidance: Working Online.* Lutterworth: BACP.

Carroll, M. (2008). Supervision and transformational learning. Available online at: www.supervisioncentre.com/docs/kv/supervision_and_transformational_learning.pdf.

Clark, M. C. (1993). Transformational learning. *New Directions for Adult and Continuing Education 57: 47–56.*

Daloz, L. A. (1999). *Mentor: Guiding the Journey of Adult Learners.* Hoboken, NJ: Wiley.

Follett, M. P. (1924). *Creative Experience.* London: Longmans Green.

Gilbert, M. C. & Evans, K. (2000). *Psychotherapy Supervision: An Integrated Relational Approach to Psychotherapy Supervision.* Buckingham: Open University Press.

Hawkins, P. & Shohet, R. (2012). *Supervision in the Helping Professions (4th edn).* Berkshire: McGraw-Hill.

Lapworth, P., Sills, C., & Fish, S. (2006). *Integration in Counselling & Psychotherapy.* London: Sage.

Roth, T. & Hill, A. (2014). *Telephone and E-Counselling Competences.* Lutterworth: BACP.

Stokes, A. (2016). *Telephone and E-Counselling Training Curriculum.* Lutterworth: BACP.

Taylor, E. W. (1998). Transformative learning: A critical review. *ERIC Clearinghouse on Adult, Career, & Vocational Education (Information Series No. 374).*

Chapter 5

New models of online supervision – (2) Breaking news! Face-to-face supervision and online supervision are not the same!!

Suzie Mosson

The FORUM model of online supervision

Professor Petruska Clarkson (1998) is quoted as saying:

> "Unlearn" to let go of the past, in order to experience the creativity and innovation that comes with trying to maintain a balance while taking advantage of the excitement of living and developing "at the edge of chaos".

Developing online supervision requires some unlearning, a lot of excitement and at times, chaos is featured, with supervisors finding themselves too close to the edge. This paper will describe FORUM. This is a model, based on the Petruska Clarkson (2008) five relationship model, adapted for use in online supervision by myself. This was initially presented to a group of peers in December 2015 and I have used it to inform my practice as a qualified online supervisor.

Several supervision models and practices have emerged alongside the growing field of counselling and therapy. Practitioners come from a variety of theoretical persuasions, although still mainly from the main historical influences of psychodynamic, behavioural, cognitive, and humanist therapy with many therapists blending different approaches as needed for specific client's needs (Carroll, 2007). In a much shorter time span, the growth of the internet and its subsequent embracement as a tool for use by the therapeutic world has created a need for faltering first steps into creating robust models for online supervision (Ainsworth, 2002).

Many experts (Bernard & Goodyear, 2004; Carroll, 2007) have struggled to explain exactly what supervision is, so what is it not? Supervision is not counselling, yet it shares many therapeutic elements, being a confidential space to offload, gain support and knowledge. Supervision is not about management; however not only is the supervisor regarded as gatekeeper and required to continually assess the supervisee – may even have to report on them – but they are often allocated by an organisation and not personally chosen. Supervision is not training, but the supervisee may seek information, references, research, and learn from the experience of the supervisor. Supervision is not about power, yet the experience differential must be acknowledged and in organisational supervision, who gets paid? Often only the supervisor since the counsellor is giving their time for free in voluntary settings.

Whether we define supervision as a working reflective alliance where feedback and guidance regarding attitude, skills and knowledge on therapeutic work can be sought (Bond 2016) or as support for an experiential and cognitive level developing skill, education, and identity (Loganbill, Hardy, & Delworth, 1982) it has become viewed as essential in some helping professions such as education, support work, nursing, ministry, and social work in the United Kingdom. It's a privileged position with responsibility for clients, counsellors, and the counselling profession as a whole.

Supervision models and theories were developed in order to give a framework to the complex interactions in supervision. Some are based on a specific theory which reflects that practised by the supervisor and supervisee; some are developmental in that the stage of the counsellor is assessed and consideration is given when offering feedback. Systems supervision focuses on the centrality of the supervisory relationship and integrated supervision draws from any number of theories and models, bringing a depth to the work which may not have been there when using a single theory (Carroll, 2007). There are really too many models to mention; however, some models have thrived and their authors are readily recognised and quoted and some have gone out of favour. The focus has moved from supervision which was rooted entirely in a counselling model, for example, purely psychoanalytic, to the reflective but still evolving frameworks offered today (Page & Wosket, 2001). Language has also evolved from the original psychoanalytic models to include unfamiliar words such as matrix, functions, tasks, dimensions and foci.

It is relevant to point out that we don't outgrow the need for supervision but continue to benefit, no matter our personal experience, skills and training. FORUM feels suitable whatever the age and stage of the online supervisee.

Platforms for change

Online technology has progressed at a much greater speed than many could have imagined. Its development has overtaken that of the radio and television and in just a fraction of the time (Gov.uk, 2014). In 2013, eighty-nine per cent of young people (Durbin, 2011) were said to access the internet via a smart phone or tablet and the maturity and acceptance of distance communication in this way has brought both benefits and pitfalls to the therapeutic counsellor. The possibility of reaching clients in need of therapy wherever they are in the world is now a reality, and supervising those same professionals in a collaborative and professionally competent way a necessity. Ideally, the technology would simply be beneath the work, supporting it; however, the reality is that attention must be paid to the impact of technology (Mulhauser, 2014) to make best and ethical use.

Counselling and supervision online can be carried out asynchronously and synchronously. Simply put, this means they may engage in a therapeutic or supervisory relationship via email which has a time delay or a video platform which allows for a conversation either in text, by voice or inclusive of a video picture as well.

The Association for Counselling and Therapy Online (ACTO) was formed in 2006 to set and maintain high standards for online counselling. Their code of ethics is in addition to a therapist's regulatory body and expects all counsellors will have regular supervision "preferably with an online supervisor" (2015). Ethics seem to be apace with online technology, but may always be a step behind due to the speed of developments online. Guidelines and encouragements are protecting both clients and therapists but what about this in online supervision?

Looking to the most recent information cascaded by the British Association of Counselling and Psychotherapy (BACP) (Bond 2015) it is considered desirable to have supervision in the method of communication the counselling took place. This additional guidance builds on that offered by Anthony and Goss (2009) who encouraged both online training and supervision. The telephone and e-counselling competences (BACP, 2015) draw attention to disinhibition, how the written word can impact, fantasy via transference in addition to trolling and catfishing (causing deliberate internet discord and using a false identity respectively) and assessing psychological and technical suitability to create and maintain an online therapeutic relationship. Risk, holding boundaries and managing a good ending are all included before supervision is mentioned. The long list of areas of competence suggests some more thought is due to be given to developing or adapting a model for online supervision. The existing models, robust though they are, did not envision the change to our world and the new competencies counsellors may be required to hold.

Using the colourful metaphor of a loom and weaving (Stokes, 2013); the models, tasks, maps, and functions of my learning plus my own and online supervisee's experiences have created and informed a way of supervising and my subsequent online supervision model is shared here. Working using both our self, as professionals and with technology it makes sense to be aware of how each impact on the other.

I work with complex and challenging couple relationships and many of my supervisees do the same: but not all of them. Some work with children and young people and some only with individual adults. I have supervisees who use mainly cognitive behavioural therapy, some who are transpersonal and some who identify as integrative. What they all have in common is that experience of complicated relationships being brought into counselling, whether it is online or in the room.

Getting to know Petruska

Professor Petruska Clarkson was a consultant psychologist, prolific writer and lecturer within the field of counselling and psychotherapy. Those who knew her personally described her as mischievous, highly creative and thought provoking. It sounds as if she was inherently human and she left a huge legacy of work when she died in 2006. In the last months and years, I have spent a great deal of time in her company and it feels a loss I never got to meet her in person.

The five-relationship model is based on the philosophical idea of intersubjectivity. This is described by Oxford Dictionary as: "Existing between conscious minds; shared by more than one conscious mind." Counselling Tutor (2013) explains this to mean shared attunement or empathy, being present and having a shared intention when looking at a relationship.

The five relationships Clarkson refers to are:

- The working alliance
- The transferential/countertransferential relationship
- The reparative/developmentally needed relationship
- The person-to-person relationship
- The transpersonal relationship

This integrated approach embraces the understanding that not all clients are the same and they do not need or want the same outcome from therapy. All these relationships may be going on at the same time or even from session to session. However, this framework felt right when going forward with online supervision in mind.

I am not a theorist; I work from experience; therefore, have peppered this paper with small examples of my work. In all cases identifying details have been changed in order to maintain confidentiality.

FORUM as a model

The adaptation of the Clarkson model to FORUM begins with the Foundation to the process of supervising online. The foundation will hold the process together if the material becomes tricky and the relationship between online supervisee and online supervisor unsteady. To create a solid foundation there should be clear contracting. Time invested in the roles and responsibilities of both online supervisee and online supervisor is never time lost. Revisiting the contract can happen at any time and is an integral part of reviewing the relationship. Exploring online etiquette is an extra dimension that face-to-face supervisors seldom have to give thought to but this, in addition to addressing which video platform, which email programme and what to do in the event of a technological difficulty are all integral facets of an online supervisory contract. Client and supervisee confidentiality, including ethics and law, must also be considered and acted on for protection of the client and also protection of the profession (ICO, 2016).

The next facet of my model is Online transference. This refers to feelings around the client noticed by both the counsellor & the supervisor. There may be fantasy and projection and they may be both positive and negative and often felt stronger via the medium of text with ro aural cues (Suler, 2007). It is psychologically useful to notice how the client distorts our own thinking and feeling and we turn from being neutral to sad, happy or angry as the session progresses. We might notice this as words, turns of phrases and metaphors that resonate from the past. This part of the relationship can be said to exist in the mind in addition to what's in the room as both transference and insight. This is particularly useful when considering the different levels of counsellor competency and also the levels of technological competency which supervisees may have. When thinking of parallel process, in particular, the parallel may include what is happening technologically. This may be attending sessions late and not allowing for program update time or sending emails without attachments, either in error or with the work written in the body of the email. The patterns give us insight. This part of the relationship is self-reflective and self-monitoring.

By reviewing development and filling the gap of knowledge, the reparative/developmental relationship identified by Clarkson can be further identified as Restorative for online supervision. The Restorative aspect of the model includes core conditions, competencies and the continual personal development (CPD) noted by Ash (1995) when exploring metaphors used by supervisees. The supervisor affirms good work, offers support & signposting and encourages reading, resources, CPD, and at times psychological education. A supervisor skilled in online working (rather than one who does it now and again) will have become adept at demonstrating nodding, apprehension and a range of emotions via email. When using a webcam it can be helpful to say, "I'm listening carefully now" after check-in to reinforce what may not be immediately obvious on a screen. The Internal supervisor prompts questions such as, "What would my supervisor say?" and offers containment. In therapy, this aspect is a safe, secure and supportive relationship intended to heal past traumas and be our adult selves. In online

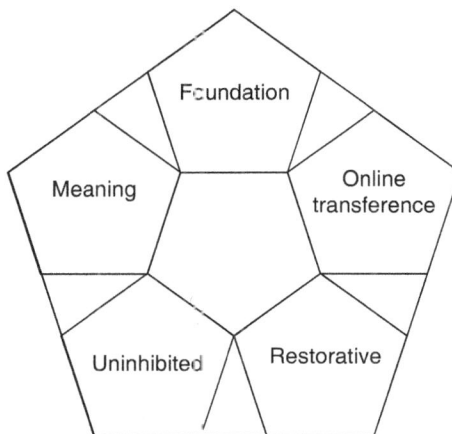

Figure 5.1 FORUM model of online supervision

supervision, it can be seen as a place where it's ok to express negative thoughts and express not knowing.

An essential part of the relationship is having the capacity for intimacy and sharing which brings us to the Uninhibited relationship. By taking part in a person-to-person relationship and bringing self into the work the online supervisor can facilitate for when something big happens in the supervisee's life. This may be because they have crossed a line boundary-wise, have a personal issue impacting on work, experienced erotic transference or have technological/confidentiality. Without confidence in the person-to-person or uninhibited relationship, it may be difficult or impossible to get through it.

Alternatively, by bringing personal issues, in particular with trainee counsellors or in new relationships, the supervisee allows for the focus to be taken from the work that is being carried out. A fabulous way of avoiding supervision where the clinical work is under the microscope! That's not to say that it's not appropriate to address these issues but this part of the relationship is highlighting the need to acknowledge and manage the supervisees needs. Opting for online supervision by webcam with a normally face-to-face practitioner may be another flag that work is being avoided. The online supervisor needs to be alert to changes in presentation for cues which suggest this (Mattinson, 1975). Power comes into play in this relationship in that supervisors are constantly evaluating and assessing and it's helpful if they take the lead in identifying what is going well or not in this facet of the relationship. Part of the power is holding the boundary between supervision and therapy and knowing when space must be made for both, whilst keeping the focus on how the therapeutic need may affect the client's process.

The final aspect of this model comes under the heading of Meaning. Carroll (1998) posited that in order to test your supervisee about beliefs they may or may not recognise, see how they feel about poking fun at slogans or dogmas. The transpersonal relationship is both the essence and value of the supervisee. Some supervisees have strong belief systems which they bring to the session. Faith, interpreting dreams, yoga, perhaps tapping may come under this. This is the soul and spirit in the session and in the participants where growth emerges from.

When presenting this model for peer scrutiny the author found it to be accepted by the group. The simplicity (yet complexity) of the model with an appropriate technological acronym was noted to be easily remembered and understood. The heart of Clarkson's work (1998, cited in Peltu, 2013) was also retained. Relationships may not be good on all fronts. Some of that will be dynamics, competence, transference or simply internet connection; however, recognising where the balance needs work allows for further depth to the supervision process.

Under the spotlight

The following snapshots of supervising online are anonymised and a combination of different supervisees, clients and pieces of work. The aim of the vignettes is to encourage curiosity and creative thinking, rather than offer them up as examples of good practice.

Foundation can be laid by using a written contract as a basis for further discussion. In addition to different contact details in the case of technology issues I find it useful to offer my personal telephone number in addition to my professional one When Fiona, a support worker, called me as needing a session between appointments she was able to contact me sooner and we were able to explore some of her anxieties immediately. This made for a more reflective online session later in the day.

Mary worked mainly in private practice and her web cam session was largely focussed on the heavy online transference involving sadness and hopelessness she experienced with a client. Prompted by a recent supervision session I had had myself, I encouraged her to remove her shoes and throw them out the room. We explored the freedom of bare feet and the casting off of her workwear, plus how she could change shoes between sessions to leave the heavy energy outside her therapy room.

The "restorative" facet of the relationship reminds me of an early experience supervising online. I observed Angela stroke her cat that she held tightly in her arms throughout her web cam session. I noticed and shared how my eye was drawn to the constant movement and how it was both distracting and comforting. I wondered some more about the cat's role for Angela and she shared her partner had moved out and she also was somewhat distracted. This allowed for checking out of support and keeping herself and clients safe.

Julie, an experienced couple counsellor, expressed by email feeling clumsy while offering mindfulness for relaxation when working online but was keen to do so. We arranged to meet on camera for our next session and by having a hot drink to hand and were able to practice using that for a mindfulness exercise. Julie allowed herself to be vulnerable and unknowing and the uninhibited element allowed for this small sharing of knowledge.

Lastly, the Meaning aspect of the relationship brings to mind Martha, a transpersonal therapist who often used email. It was at the time of Brexit, that being the colloquial term for Britain leaving the European Union. Martha had experienced a similar situation in her home country which had led to violence and unrest on the street where she lived and she was fearful of the same happening where she now lived. I had no answers or experience and shared I was at ease with the not knowing, unlike herself, and we continued to explore what it meant for not just her, but also for the clients she would see. Additionally, we were able to acknowledge how her personal experience gave her greater understanding when we considered the countries some of her clients came from.

As online therapy and supervision have gained respect due to its increasing availability, safety, and flexibility, the models we use must adapt to meet the challenge. The future of online supervision is an ongoing learning process and this model is not the end of the road any more than the end of the information highway.

References

ACTO (2015). *Professional Conduct and Code of Ethics.* Available online at: www.acto-uk.org/professional-conduct-code-of-ethics/.

Ainsworth, M. (2002). *E-Therapy: History and Survey Development of E-Therapy from 1972–2002.* Available online at: www.metanoia.org/imhs/history.htm.

Anthony, K., & Goss, S. (2009). *Guidelines for Online Counselling and Psychotherapy including Guidelines for Online Supervision (3rd edn).* Lutterworth: British Association for Counselling & Psychotherapy.

Ash, E. (1995). Supervision: Taking account of feelings. In: J. Pritchard (Ed.), *Good Practice in Supervision, Statutory and Voluntary Organisations.* London: Jessica Kingsley.

BACP (2015). BACP: Research. Available online at: www.bacp.co.uk/research/competences/. Accessed 23 September 2016, only available to BACP members.

Bernard, J. M., & Goodyear, R. K. (2004). *Fundamentals of Clinical Supervision (3rd edn).* Boston, MA: Pearson.

Bond, T. (2015). *Good Practice in Action 047: Ethical Framework for the Counselling Professions Supplementary Guidance: Working Online.* Lutterworth: BACP.

Bond, T. (2016). *Ethical Framework for the Counselling Professions.* Lutterworth: BACP.

Carroll, M. (1998). *Spirituality, values and supervision.* Keynote address, British Association for Supervision Practice and Research. Third International Conference on Supervision, St Mary's College, Strawberry Hill.

Carroll, M. (2007). One More Time – What is Supervision? *Psychotherapy in Australia, 13(3):* 34–40.

Clarkson, P. (2008). *The Therapeutic Relationship (2nd edn).* London: Whurr. Available online at: http://web.archive.org/web/20061006235927/http://www.psych.lse.ac.uk/complexity/Seminars/1998/clarkson98jan.htm

Counselling Tutor (2013). Petruska Clarkson – 5 relationship model explained. Available online at: www.youtube.com/watch?v=V-E1Uxw7d_g#t=11.

Durbin, C. (2011). Internet & mobility: Youth technology trends. *Technology Trends Report.* Available online at: www.saferinternet.org.uk/research/additional-resources.

Government Digital Inclusion Strategy – Gov.uk (2014). Available online at: www.gov.uk/government/publications/government-digital-inclusion-strategy/government-digital-inclusion-strategy.

Information Commissioners Office (2016). *Information security, Principle 7.* Available online at: *https://ico.org.uk/for-organisations/guide-to-data-protection/principle-7-security/.*

Intersubjective (2016). In: *OxfordDictionaries.com.* Available online at: https://en.oxforddictionaries.com/definition/intersubjective.

Loganbill, C., Hardy, E., & Delworth, U. (1982). Supervision: A conceptual model. *Counseling Psychologist, 10:* 3–42.

Peltu, M. (2013). *Clarkson's Presentation – January 1998.* Available online at: www.lse.ac.uk/researchAndExpertise/units/complexity/Seminars/1998/clarkson98jan.aspx.

Mattinson, J. (1975). *The Reflection Process in Casework Supervision.* London: Tavistock Institute of Marital Studies.

Mulhauser, G. (2014). Disadvantages of Counselling or Therapy by Email. Available online at: http://counsellingresource.com/therapy/service/online-disadvantages/.

Page, S., & Wosket, V. (2001). *Supervising the Counsellor: A Cyclical Model (2nd edn).* London: Routledge.

Stokes, A. (2013). The warp and weft of online supervision. *TILT Magazine – Therapeutic Innovations in Light of Technology 13:* 49. Available online at: http://issuu.com/onlinetherapyinstitute/docs/tiltissue13/49.

Suler, J. (2007). The psychology of text relationships. *The Psychology of Cyberspace.* Available online at: http://users.rider.edu/~suler/psycyber/psytextrel.html.

Chapter 6

New models of online supervision – (3) CARER

Liane Collins

Page and Woskett argue that the most important piece of equipment for any supervisor is a conceptual understanding or model of supervision (Page & Woskett, 2001). When I started my diploma course in online therapeutic supervision I had done no previous supervisory work, other than in a tutoring capacity. I had no idea about supervisory models or that I would be integrating models from a variety of fields to build my own. However, only a few months later, a number of supervision sessions, and much reading and discussion, I started to find my own voice and way of working online. This chapter describes my learning from established models and the personal processing that delivered me finally to my own working model of supervision.

> Models help me to clarify what I do in supervision. Models guide us and give us a sense of what we are doing and why. Without that clarity supervision would be aimless, and may be unhelpful and ineffective. (van Ooijen, 2003)

Background

I feel that my model of online supervision began many years ago. I have been through a number of incarnations in my working life, the first being nurse training at eighteen years old and, although it was now a long time ago, this was obviously so indoctrinated that I continued to use the principals taught then all through my teaching career and still use them now. The model of working utilises the elements of the nursing process – assess, plan, implement, evaluate – in conjunction with Roper, Logan, and Tierney's (1983) "activities of living" model in a problem-solving manner.

I then began the teaching part of my career. Using the above to guide my work I added thinking, relating, creating, communicating, which make use of the elements of the teaching process. This should lead those who are motivated to inquire, infer, and interpret; to think reflectively, critically and creatively; and to make use of the knowledge and skills they have gained by becoming effective decision makers. Similarly, objective, instruction, evaluation linked by understanding and motivation is the Gage and Berliner teaching and learning model mantra, (McIlrath & Huitt, 1995), and is based on the teacher's knowledge of students' characteristics and how best to motivate them.

The combination of these models then builds the foundation for my current model of online supervision.

Kuntze, van der Molen, and Born (2009) identified seven basic counselling communication skills:

- minimal encouragements
- asking questions
- paraphrasing
- reflection of feeling
- concreteness
- summarising
- situation clarification

And five advanced skills, which also form part of my online synchronous and asynchronous communication with my supervisees. They are:

- advanced accurate empathy
- confrontation
- positive re-labelling
- examples of one's own
- directness

Assessment of the supervisee and their developmental level, qualification, experience and area of working helps to determine their proficiency or competency in their field. In addition, it opens areas for potential further professional development. Determining their objective for supervision also ensures that I will have the competency to work with them and issues relevant to their practice.

Planning relates first to a formal written agreement between us, ensuring that we both work within an ethical and legal framework and are entering the supervisory relationship with as much information as possible regarding our working arrangements. The contract should suit the supervisee's needs and stage of counselling development. Using a model creates clear boundaries for supervision work and can be related to the stage of the supervisee. Setting objectives and planning may also be part of each individual session, making sure all necessary areas are given appropriate time and attention.

In online practice, there is the necessity to add other features to this contract that would not be required for in-the-room work. Technology can occasionally be tricky and, to reduce anxiety, it is necessary to have a plan b and both to have an appreciation that this can happen. A shared mobile phone number can offer an opportunity for text if things go wrong online. Holding emails can be sent so your supervisee knows you have received their communication and when you will respond in full. Consideration needs to be given to encryption and password protecting documents that could be accessed by others, and also storage of these communications. When working and talking about clients, all information should be anonymous and full client communications should not be sent to the supervisor. Working online also needs to be covered by data protection and the holder of personal data needs to be registered with the Information Commissioner's Office.

Implementation and Instruction form the basis of each session with thinking, relating, creating, communicating, understanding and motivation being the underpinning of this part of supervision time.

Each session, and the supervisory relationship as a whole, end in evaluation – to review and reflect on the content and consider next steps. This may then return to assessment and setting of objectives, or, within a session, informing the moving on to the next issue, forming not so much a cyclical, but more of a spiral containment for the supportive working relationship.

This brings us to the 'filling' – the integration of supervisory models that inform my practice.

My approach to supervision has developed, and will continue to develop, in stages and is influenced by technological development and understanding, my reading and research into supervision and by reflecting on and reviewing my practice as a supervisor, both in person and online. I have explored many established f2f models of supervision, each emphasising a different focus, in an endeavour to develop an integrated, but meaningful model for online supervision.

My most recent mantra is restorative, formative, normative. This Inskipp and Proctor (1993) process model trio is what sits now in my mind as I work.

Here is where the tasks and functions of supervision lead to the process – the tasks being counselling skills development, professional role, emotional awareness, and self-evaluation, and the functions of monitoring and evaluating, advising, modelling, exploring, and supporting. Much of supervision takes place where these functions and tasks intermingle. In the broader landscape of the language, it allows for diversity and difference in counselling backgrounds and in models and theoretical approaches. The model feels simple but effective, describing the full experience of the supervisory relationship – that is: considering the inherent features which involve exploration, support, recharge, and confidence; quality assurance, monitoring of standards, and responsibility; understanding, awareness and facilitation of the dynamic. The restorative and formative parts sit with the models I already knew and followed and normative brings in the necessary professional element.

The scientific approach of the discrimination model of supervision developed by Bernard and Goodyear (as cited in Leddick, 2001) – observation, evaluation, facilitation, and problem solving – appealed to me straight away as a psychology graduate and a science teacher. It seemed to be designed to build on strengths and focus on talents, encouraging self-efficacy. It also involved the three roles of Counsellor (restorative), teacher (formative) and consultant (normative). Fitting neatly for me with Inskipp and Proctor (1993), as cited in Henderson (2001).

The counsellor role identifies unresolved issues that potentially cloud the therapeutic relationship. It helps supervisees notice their blind spots or where they are "hooked" by a client's issues. The consultant is an ethical role, like the normative process, to ensure good and balanced practice. The teacher role is used to build skills in the supervisee. This skill building is also split into three parts. *Process* is how communication is conveyed and whether the supervisee is reflecting the client's emotions. "Conceptualisation" helps the supervisee to explain their application of a specific theory to a case they are bringing to supervision, seeing the bigger picture, and exploring what might be done next and why. "Personalisation" is the supervisee's use of self in the supervision session. The aim is that all involved are non-defensively present in the relationship. I felt this model would especially meet the needs of a trainee counsellor or supervisor on the lower levels of development and competence.

The cyclical model of Page and Wosket (2001) is structured with contract, focus, space, bridge, review, and seems to me to fill all the previous criteria of assessing, planning and objective, in line with the initial normative stage of counselling agreements (see also chapter three). The space offers the restorative thinking, relating, creating – well, implementation of space! The bridge brings us back to the task in hand – the work with the supervisee directly and their relationship with the client indirectly, and the understanding, communicating and motivation involved in the instructive and formative elements of supervision. The process is finalised by evaluation and review. A much-abbreviated version by Hawkins and Shohet (2012) describes these same supervision process stage elements with the terminology reflection, exploration, focus, reflection as does their acronym CLEAR – contract, listen, explore, action, review.

Stages are met through each session and throughout the relationship. They may become more spiral in nature and also cross back and forth between stages. In addition, not all may be met within a session, depending on the needs of the supervisee, but all will be connected with over time.

However, the Hawkins and Shohet seven-eyed model in my opinion is very dependent on the relationship and seeing someone in the room and so some adaptation to the way of thinking may be needed to adopt it to online work. It also seems to me that certain assumptions may be made about the client who is not present. There appears to be a focus on the client where the supervisee is being asked to stand in the client's shoes, which then becomes what the supervisee assumes and recalls – to then inform the supervisor's interpretation – a bit like Chinese whispers. There seems to be something false about that extra step. I am also aware that I struggle with its reliance on transference and counter transference. As a person-centred counsellor, I only have a vague idea of the concept and wonder if this is really what I would just call empathy. The developers of this model specifically claim its ability to meet diverse issues and needs, which no doubt it does, but I would also assert that PC models cover this at a foundation level with the core values of empathy, understanding and non-judgement for all with the addition of gentle curiosity.

I am very keen on creative counselling and so following on, creative supervision. In my previous counselling work with children in schools and in training with the Place2Be, we encouraged the use of play for expression and used creativity in the supervision room as the third space. This is heavily influenced by the developmental psychological practice of Lev Vygotsky (1962), and therapeutic distance. It also offers opportunities for therapeutic story writing, the use of puppets, and metaphor to consider and possibly change ways of thinking. There is immense therapeutic value in the application of modelling in sand tray work and Play Doh to help supervisees understand the relationships they have with their clients, how their clients respond in therapy and how therapy aims can be visualised for follow through. I'm not sure how many supervisees would be open to trying it unless they used the techniques already with children. It is a model that also requires imagination to apply to an online environment, and some understanding of technology, but video in addition to text can make supervision with creative methods interesting and thought provoking; drawing and painting apps can be shared, as can virtual whiteboards such as WebWhiteBoard, RealtimeBoard or Scribblar.

Finally, the over-arching "icing on the cake". My initial counselling training was person-centred and this approach colours my current online supervisory work. In practicing the core conditions of Roger's person-centred model (2004) – congruency, unconditional positive regard and empathy – in the online supervisory sessions, I trust that this modelling of working will influence the supervisee's work with their client.

Rogers (2004) introduced the concept of actualisation, potentially freeing the supervisor to trust in the work of the supervisee with their client, and in the client's ability to make the best use of the work. The supervisor does not need to monitor or assess, or generally police, the work of the supervisee and so can concentrate on helping the supervisee to explore their own thoughts and ideas about their work. An important note to consider is the legal and ethical standpoint. The BACP guidelines (Bond, 2015) suggest supervisors have ethical, though not legal, guidelines, and regarding clients there is an emphasis on the responsibilities of the supervisee/counsellor, but not the supervisor. They also refer to requirements rather than responsibilities. This suggests the supervisory relationship is more a mutual than hierarchical one and defers responsibility for the client to the counsellor.

Rogers developed his theory for counselling, not for supervision, and it was developed from experience in his practice. This involved the nature of the human organism, a theory of personality, a theory of the fully functioning organisation, a theory of interpersonal relationship, and the theoretical implications for various human activities. Tudor and Worrall (2004) suggest, that in the process of supervision, the theory of personality sits at the centre of thinking as the condition under which we develop patterns of thought and behaviour, and that supervision is based on a theory of therapy including its conditions, process and outcomes.

This reminds us we have the capacity to be congruent and unselfconscious – though this may be easier said than done. We have all developed ideas about how we should be in the world and what we should be or do in order to be accepted by others. We therefore have things that we have difficulty in acknowledging or articulating accurately – perhaps feelings we suspect will not be acceptable – which may limit our work. During training and our work as counsellors we start out perhaps untrained but not unskilled, but over time we develop new conditions of worth related to our concept of ourselves as therapists and practitioners – a professional self-concept – which can limit our behaviour as counsellors and supervisors. There are echoes here of Robinson's (1974) developmental stage model of competence.

Regular online reviews throughout the process maintain focus on my supervisee's needs and help me to consider my role in relation to their normative, formative, restorative and also their changing needs throughout the relationship.

The differing, but similar, aspects of proficiency and competence confused me until discussion with my course tutor. Competence implies a minimum level of skill, while proficient implies expertise or mastery. It seems to me that I need to be proficient in the area in which I am working, and so my starting point must be the area in which I have most training and experience. Further training is then required to suit the idiosyncrasies of the online work; so, in my situation, training and experience online is vital to understanding the discrete nature and subtle differences this way of working brings to counselling. The ability to make use of and read with understanding text-based material and respond with warmth and acceptance without access to other visual, aural or oral cues is vital.

The BACP Supplementary Guidance for Working Online (Bond, 2015) recommends making use of online supervision, thus ensuring that in my reflection that I am working competently and gaining proficiency in my practice. Personally, I believe that online supervision should be mandatory for online counselling. I have further evidence for this from my online counselling courses and work, as well as teaching as an online tutor with students, delivering courses, and managing tutorials, with general supervisory support through their role-play situations as client and counsellor. While we may approach supervision from different, or even integrated, models, I feel we function more effectively if we work within a theory whose principles are comparable to our own personal philosophy.

Professional online supervision is a significant source of my learning and support, and so should be for my own supervisees. Working within the domains of influence allows the practitioner and supervisor to understand the context in which the practice takes place. This allows the supervisor congruently to offer appropriate empathic understanding to the supervisees work. The ability to offer congruence, understanding, and acceptance to a supervisee's work is essential to the supervision relationship. Power and responsibility are shared more equitably between the supervisor and supervisee. Based on a person-centred model, self-awareness and personal understanding are built through the process, tasks and relationship. I am aware I want to "fix" things but I must appreciate that my supervisee is a professional practitioner in their own right, and that they are responsible for their client. Understanding then may be developed through triangulation of interaction and previous experience.

My favoured online approach is based on this person-centred working alliance with my own supervisor's preferred practice of collaborative dialogue (Anderson, 1997) playing a major part, where the learning style of the supervisee is taken into account. In my personal supervision, I have the advantage of learning from modelled practice and being in a relationship where my supervisor also has the knowledge and experience of the unique nature of online work.

However, all the approaches discussed here have their influence and play their own part. I see each model as offering ways of thinking and working that can be effectively integrated according to the issue brought by the online supervisee based on their individual learning style. This integrative approach can be used in all current main platforms of online supervision – email, Skype, or other more appropriate HIPAA/HITECH- compliant voice, video and screen sharing software, and in the use of a whiteboard. Additionally, online supervision and the inherent creativity of narrative can develop the supervisee's self-awareness, offering emotional and restorative support and overlapping in some ways with the role of personal therapy.

So where am I in terms of my model for online supervision? Well it's all of this, though many overlap. What I notice about all of these models is that I do bits of each of them. If I deconstruct my sessions, I can plot them against all the models, though in practice I am not actively thinking about them during the session. In that respect, it is different from counselling.

Being fond of acronyms I would describe my personal model as relationship, assess, creatively express, review, but RACER does not seem an appropriate acronym to suit a supervisory relationship. Instead, perhaps I will describe it as CARER – contract, assess, relationship, explore/educate, review; five small words, with the relationship at the core, which encompass, I hope, the two and a half thousand words that precede them.

References

Anderson, H. (1997). *Conversation, Language, and Possibilities: A Post-Modern Approach to Therapy*. New York: Basic Books.

Bond, T. (2015). *Good Practice in Action 047: Ethical Framework for the Counselling Professions Supplementary Guidance: Working Online.* Lutterworth: BACP.

Hawkins, P. & Shohet, R. (2012). *Supervision in the Helping Professions (4th edn)*. Berkshire: McGraw-Hill.

Henderson, P. (2001). Supervision and the mental health of the counsellor. In: M. Carroll & M. Tholstrup (Eds.), *Integrative Approaches to Supervision* (pp. 93–107). London: Jessica Kingsley.

Inskipp, F., & Proctor, B. (1993). *The Art, Craft & Tasks of Counselling Supervision*. Twickenham: Cascade.

Kuntze, J., van der Molen, H., & Born, M. P. (2009). Increase in counselling communication skills after basic and advanced microskills training. *British Journal of Educational Psychology, 79(1)*: 175–188.

Leddick, G. R. (2001). supervision models. *CYC Online, 24.* Available online at: www. cyc-net.org/cyc-online/cycol-0101-supervision%20models.html.

McIlrath, D. & Huitt, W. (1995). The teaching-learning process: A discussion of models. *Educational Psychology Interactive.* Valdosta, GA: Valdosta State University. Available online at: www.edpsycinteractive.org/papers/modeltch.html.

Ooijen van, E. (2003). *Clinical Supervision Made Easy: The 3-Step Method.* London: Churchill Livingstone.

Page, S. & Wosket, V. (2001). *Supervising the Counsellor: A Cyclical Model.* Hove: Routledge.

Robinson, O. (1974). *Conscious Competence Learning Model.* Available online at: www. businessballs.com.

Rogers, C. R. (2004). *On Becoming a Person: A Therapist's View of Psychotherapy.* London: Constable and Robinson.

Roper, Logan, & Tierney. (1983). *Activities of Living.* Royal College of Nursing archive 2004. Available online at: www.rcn.org.uk/development/learning/transcultural_health/ transcultural/adulthealth/sectionthree

Tudor, K. & Worrall, M. (2004). *Freedom to Practice: Person-Centred Approaches to Supervision.* Ross-on-Wye: PCCS Books.

Vygotsky, L. S. (1962). *Thought and Language.* E. Hanfmann & G. Vakar (Trans.). Cambridge, MA: MIT & Wiley.

Chapter 7

Evaluating online supervision relationship and process

Suzie Mosson

> *O wad some Pow'r the giftie gie us
> To see oursels as others see us
> It wad frae monie a blunder free us
> An' foolish notion
> What airs in dress an' gait wad lea'e us
> An' ev'n Devotion
> > (Burns, probably written
> > late in 1785)[1]

As online counselling has started to move to the mainstream, online supervision practice is now beginning to flourish. This chapter will be based around FORUM, the adapted Petruska Clarkson (1990) relationship model that I devised for supervising online (see chapter five for a more detailed account). The variances between face-to-face supervision and that delivered online revealed themselves during clinical practice and have been explored both reflectively and critically with peers on a small scale. FORUM continues to be a developing but simple model which can be used as a framework by the contemporary membership of professional online supervisors and those emerging from training and developing their personal way of working therapeutically online. These few words are not a "to do list", but to encourage reflection and open discussion around the valuable multi-faceted relationship between online counsellors and their supervisors. A relationship often viewed with envy by other professionals who work in a therapeutic way with clients.

Figure 7.1 displays a pentagon enclosing five key relationships balanced and fitting together perfectly. You can see foundation, online transference, restorative, uninhibited, and meaning relationships slotting together to be drawn on at different times in the sessions. This parallels and links closely to Clarkson's own model which speaks of the working alliance, the transferential relationship, the reparative relationship, the real (or person to person) relationship and the transpersonal relationship (Counselling Tutor, 2013).

In my view, all aspects of FORUM are necessary. They allow addressing of process, tasks and include stages of online supervision. Realistically, perfect online

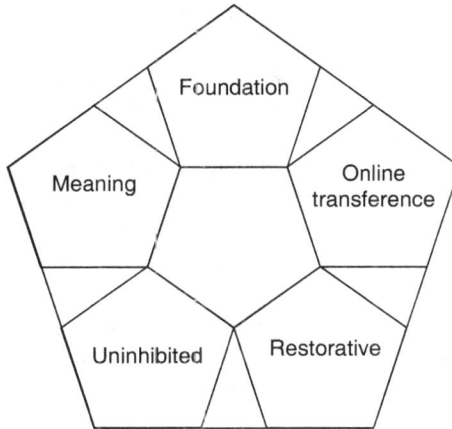

Figure 7.1 FORUM model of online supervision

supervision sessions are not often attained, if ever; however, through evaluating our performance as online supervisors and collaborating with online supervisees and others our supervision work online can be robustly informed.

Liz Beddoe, a trainer and researcher who was visiting and teaching in Scotland from New Zealand delivered a hugely interesting seminar at my local university (2015Beddoe 2015) She stated: "Never trust anybody who says 'I don't need supervision'." Her words stayed with me and I sought out the paper of the same name (Beddoe, Davys, & Adamson, 2014) as I worked my way through existing models of supervision and considered online issues which may occur. If she feels so strongly the important question must be why? In addition, is it really that important to have supervision in the same nature as the counselling is delivered?

No safety net required

First, I'll look at some of the reasons that supervisees might give for not needing supervision or covertly avoiding it. The AdEPT (Understanding and Preventing the Adverse Effects of Psychological Therapies, 2016) study found many varied and often understandable reasons for not attending supervision when looking at adverse effects which negatively affected therapy.

Sometimes counsellors can feel judged, either personally or professionally. Supervisors are people too so sometimes say clumsy things by accident. Off the cuff comments about anything from the quality of a car or dislike of a particular counselling technique can affect the motivation to attend supervision. If a supervisee is using a new or different model with a client, they may feel uneasy about taking their great success or little movement to supervision for fear of getting into trouble for working outside their field.

Unfortunately, if online supervision is text based the words can stay burned into a page which is where the importance of a collegial relationship becomes particularly important, where it's okay to disagree and check things out. It's essential that it's clear from the beginning that misunderstandings can and do happen and the only way through them is to bring them out into the open (Jones & Stokes, 2009; Munro, 2002).

Online counsellors can quickly become overcommitted either emotionally or timewise. A sudden increase of clients being slotted into every small space, increase in other workload or an illness in the family can allow the counsellor to feel they are doing just fine and supervision can wait. This conflicts with British Association of Counselling and Psychotherapy's (BACP) new ethical framework (Bond, 2016). A particular challenge when counselling online is the opportunity to continue to sit in at the workstation and linger to answer emails and research long after the session has ended thus impacting on physical health in additional to emotional wellbeing. The self-care strategies counsellors have learned along the way can become side-lined and battered by the challenging work we all do with the risk their work has become impaired and their ability to function diminished.

Neuroscience links empathy in the room to mirroring in the brain which can be detrimental to the counsellor when working in complex and challenging subjects. Lisa Jenner (2016) speaks of the impact of trauma on herself as a therapist and supervisor and how she consciously incorporates self-care during sessions and not just outside them. When reflecting on self-care perhaps we should consider supervision like mindfulness. There is a (allegedly) Zen proverb which encourages: "You should sit in meditation for twenty minutes every day — unless you're too busy. Then you should sit for an hour." I can't find the source for this but I think it's fitting and has a punch which keeps it memorable, even if it was intended as a social media meme rather than as a wise Buddhist decree.

I have a suspicion that online counsellors in private practice may be particularly drawn to fitting in "just one more" client into their diary as they may not be restricted by lack of receptionists and closing of offices when they work online. That additional flexibility that allows them to work through different time zones works against them. There may also be a parallel with the online supervisor who feels pressure from many organisational and private online supervisees vying for diary space. The pressure may not be immediately obvious as the supervisor does their best to accommodate everyone's needs and putting themselves last. Consequently, they may not be giving of their best at times.

Sadly, online counsellors who feel their personal and professional power being eroded may hesitate over making the next online supervision appointment. This may be where there has been no room for collaboration or they feel education has been withheld when requested or offered when not. Appointment arranging may be on an ad hoc basis allowing the online counsellor to fall away without notice or ending. We speak of disinhibition and our noticing of clients but practicing online professionals may also be subject to this phenomenon. The notion "you can't see me" can allow hiding in plain sight and also bring in harmful and punitive projections in some cases (Suler, 2004a).

Being kept late, finishing early, changing appointments at short notice or particularly often will all impact on the online relationship. Working online does not mean simply turning up at the appointed time but continuing to prepare in the same way as face-to-face supervision. This means ensuring the connection is strong and updates are in place so not being taken by surprise when switching on the laptop. Boundaries are just as important when on a portable device as in the therapy room when contracting (Yonan, Bardick, & Willment, 2011).

Working across countries may mean supervision is not seen as a requirement or even beneficial by the online counsellor. It may not be recognised as good practice in the country from where they work. It may come as a surprise to those of us who diligently arrange sessions, keen to download the clients they find lurking in the recesses of their minds after the session has ended, that their colleagues across the world have never been offered this gem.

In some instances, lack of suitable training can mean the online counsellor sees themselves in the role of expert and therefore having no need for supervision. Their training has finished and in the same way personal therapy may be seen as ended on graduation, supervision may be seen as an extra to dip in and out of only when things feel particularly tough. There may be many factors in making this decision but if the outcome is to withdraw from the nature of supervision, there is a lost opportunity for growth in addition to no regulation of the counsellor's work and the possibility of burn out more likely than if attending regular supervision.

The United Kingdom Council for Psychotherapy (UKCP) *Supervision Policy* (2012) specifically makes mention of burnout when outlining what they see as counsellor obligations. If the relationship becomes stuck between the online supervisor and supervisee and a crisis point has been reached where there is severe psychological stress creating burnout symptoms, Hutton (2012, p. 29) questions, "are supervisors ethical guardians or submissive observers?" He links his concerns to untrained or inexperienced supervisors who are unable to recognise the signals. The tightrope walked by some may mean they are unable to take responsibility for contracting to meet their supervisory obligations.

Firm foundations

BACP's Supplementary Guidance for Online Work, written by Professor Tim Bond (2015), are clear that when working online with clients, a parallel for at least some of the supervision should be in the same manner. Online therapeutic training has not been identified as mandatory by any of the regulatory bodies (to date) and there are few skilled and specifically qualified online supervisors to be found.

Many supervisors are working with only minimal training in online therapeutic work and this can create difficulties in ensuring that effective supervision is delivered. Some supervisors may have personal experience of being online with friends and family, either via text or video, but may not be familiar with the ethical and technological challenges their supervisee may face through working regularly with the fickle nature of the internet (Stokes & Wilson, 2015). An ability to recognise online defences may not be developed fully and they may not be able to respond empathically in a way that can be heard (Evans 2009). It's possible that vulnerable online clients may be at more risk of harm and the supervisor themselves may not be comfortable with the slightly more directive or solution focused way of working.

A quick internet search of the Association for Counselling and Therapy Online (ACTO) website who hold directories of online therapists shows many supervisors tend towards Skype for supervision sessions when working online. Used carefully this can be successful so long as both supervisor and supervisee are mindful of confidentiality. This means simple steps like ensuring passwords aren't known by others, text is deleted after sessions and no-one can overhear what is being discussed. The contents of the sessions are likely to be of little interest to anyone who has the capacity to hack into Skype and the sessions are likely to be more secure than those held by telephone; however, the need for a private space continues to be a priority.

Taking the focus back to the client, it's worth remembering that Skype identities are often shared between couples and a partner may have a vested interest in knowing the content of counselling sessions. Therefore, the online supervisor having an awareness of recording or key logging devices is helpful in addition to reminding clients that the app they are using is likely replicated on all their equipment. Other platforms such as Vsee, Zoom and FaceTime are also used by a number of online supervisors in addition to bespoke platforms used for only therapeutic work. Which platform is most suitable is not definitive and I would encourage supervisors and supervisees to do their own research in this ever-changing area. In the same way, we would not consider sharing information on a telephone party line (remember those?), now that there are alternatives it makes sense to keep up to date with technology as it evolves and the level of confidentiality required.

The nature of using the internet may find clients wanting to get straight down to business and have an expectation more in line with sourcing and buying goods online. Given the space they may step straight into the issue without preamble and possibly leave just as quickly. This may catch online counsellors by surprise when considering contracting and confidentiality and a skilled online supervisor should be able to help manage this and prevent this occurring by modelling safe steps at the beginning of the online relationship.

Encrypted or password protected emails can be used for online supervision safely in order to transfer information from one computer to another and this particular way of working can be preferable to those who work peripatetically as it allows for greater flexibility of time as well as location. The same security rules apply for passwords being safe and in addition it's worth noting that email services such as Safe-mail, Hushmail, etc., require both parties to use the same company for protection unless specific additional steps are taken. It's not just a case of email and go as some would wrongly assume and send the email only minimally protected.

A closed forum, such as used by Online Training for Counsellors Ltd (OLT) student campus, could be used for either individual or group online supervision. I have noted how, when tutoring online students, they share therapeutically when in training and at times ask for specific help of the group. If offered the opportunity to have supervision this way, there is no reason to refuse it and it may fit the needs of some who feel strongly against email or webcam/text sessions. Again, encryption and password protection allows for the safety and security as the other platforms available. There are several creative ways of working online and benefitting from online supervision, whatever your particular need or skill or talent. Ensuring the cohesive fit is the beginning of exploring alternative means of self-expression (Fenichel, et al, 2001) and it's worthwhile finding an online supervisor who understands using doodles, whiteboards or picture boards if that is part of the online counsellor's way of working with clients.

Looking at liability, not all insurance companies are comfortable with online counselling and supervision and an integral part of preparing to work online is to ensure cover is in place and adequate. Online supervisees may have restrictions on countries their clients can engage from or even restrict the format of their work. A common restriction is requiring a face-to-face meeting take place before the work begins online. This is plainly not always possible logistically as in many cases the parties may be in different countries or there may be mobility issues which prevent this. The British Insurance Brokers Association (BIBA 2016) have an awareness of this when considering data protection and are referred to by BACP (2016) on their website from which prospective clients may use to seek therapists. However, in the same way that online counsellors hold and share knowledge regarding safety and security online explicitly with their client group, the online supervisor holds this responsibility for the online supervisee. It is their responsibility to keep up to date and ensure their supervisee is taking responsibility also for their knowledge and understanding.

With these many factors to consider when creating a secure base, it feels worth remembering online supervision is therapeutic work and as such the core conditions of empathy, congruence, and unconditional positive regard continue to be necessary to underpin the work. We cannot disregard the humanness of the interactions and focus totally on the technology to its detriment.

What's it all about?

Having looked at some of the reasons counsellors and other therapeutically trained professionals don't seek out supervision it might be more helpful to look at why they do. Figure 7.2 shows some of the commonly cited reasons by supervisees in my online experience. The focus pointing to protecting clients, ensuring the work is in their best interest and making the best ethical version of ourselves as supervisors and supervisees.

This is in line with Carroll (2007); however, his historical walk through supervision makes no mention of online experiences and their place in the present.

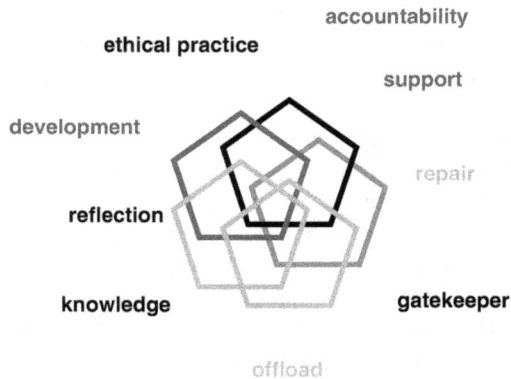

Figure 7.2 Reasons for supervision

As a note of interest, searching BACP professional conduct cases recently showed many investigations regarding counsellors. There are few live cases which refer to supervisors, and at the time of writing this, none were online supervisors. The complaints theme was around the breakdown of the supervisory relationship and I note that, in the situations researched, a dual role is often held with the supervisee. The unacknowledged significant relationships caused distress due to lack of confidentiality, abuse of power and it would seem lack of self-awareness, thus bringing about the professional conduct investigation.

Covert thoughts and feelings may even be more strongly felt in the online relationship than face-to-face sessions when we consider the disinhibition effect and strongly felt transference and countertransference (Suler, 2004b). The feeling of distance, lack of personal face-to-face relationship and the small world of counselling means there is every possibility the online supervisor/supervisee relationship *is* dual in some way. This inevitably makes the relationship more complex but not untenable. Supervision of supervision is necessary to explore the supervision work, the dynamics and where perspective may be clouded. There may be a reluctance to confront or lack of objectivity which becomes hidden behind the dual relationship and is more helpfully opened up and explored.

The aim of the two questions shown in Figure 7.3 is not to draw up another list referring to a paper or text book, but to look to ourselves. What can be offered by you that another online supervisor may not be able to offer? As supervisors are as different as snowflakes, you may recognise some of the thoughts below, perhaps in yourself.

The questions are useful to share with online supervisees. As training ends and practice develops, monitoring of their own best cases and useful methods must be established in the absence of reports to educational organisations and self-reflective papers (Feltham & Dryden, 2006).

What do your online supervisees gain from you that is a bonus?
What do your online supervisees lose by having you as a supervisor?

Figure 7.3 Self reflection

Some supervisors may be skilled in a particular model or have years of experience in a number of roles. They may have a knack for working creatively online and enthusiasm for sharing. Many online supervisors have hands on experience of accreditation processes or perhaps it's simply understanding that is a bonus. Understanding the knotty, simple or challenging queries their supervisees bring and being able to simplify the problems, breaking them down to be examined calmly and without allowing strong projections to affect the work adversely, is their skill.

An online supervisor can receive actual extracts of the work in text form (with the full agreement of the client). The writing explored in context can be unpacked and studied by the counsellor and their wonderings further explored in an online supervision session. Rhythm, typos and speed of response can be recognised. This can be a rich source of understanding and clarity and similar to the strategy of Interpersonal Process Recall developed by Kagan (1974). By using text rather than video or audio to record the session, the online supervisor has the tools to be curious and look to the covert thoughts and feeling which occurred during the session.

Changing the tone of the question to explore where personal drawbacks are when supervising online is challenging but necessary. Only by asking for and exploring this information can the shadow side be uncovered and subsequent changes made (Johnston, 2014).

Some online supervisors are quick to get to the point, not allowing space for exploration and conversely there are supervisors who never offer an opinion, their experience or direction. Synchronous text can feel slow, as if the online supervisor is not fully present, and connections late, seemingly hindered by technology breakdowns. Conversely typing can be experienced as too fast, inhibiting reflective thought as the pressure to respond equally fast builds over the session. Online supervisees may also be affected adversely when the family pet introduces themselves across the computer screen, disrupting the session in a way which would never be considered in face-to-face practice.

Humour can be offered and misread or found overbearing when in the written word. Emoji's can jar and be inaccurately interpreted and whilst often used to dispel tension, the outcome can feel harsh and triggering. Jumping up to answer the doorbell during a session, receiving cups of coffee from partners and greeting children who are returning home from school can feel diminishing to the counsellor and disrespectful to the work and relationship. These are real examples I have experienced in the online supervision role, not fabricated ideas and happen surprisingly often. In the counselling room, the supervisor has the power to make the space almost distraction free, but may feel they are without the power to do that in online role, or it may not have occurred to them that they need to be explicit. These are all learning experiences, however, and material to be explored (Yalom, 2002).

Confessional

Informal checking out during each online supervision session such as, "How was that for you?", "Was that helpful?", "Have we covered what we need to?" may be commonly asked by way of evaluation. In order to improve the sessions, or ensure they are useful, we need to seek feedback, whether it is positive of negative. We also consider what we feel has gone well (Page & Wosket, 1994). Perhaps noting where a connection has been made to theory with the supervisee, or an acknowledgement of a blind spot or giving a really affirming, "thank you so much" when preparing our next session. We may reflect on words used, changes in the relationship or responses which were out of character for the supervisee we have come to know. The first time I used a genogram via webcam with a new supervisee, I patted myself on the back, feeling the glow of the supervisee's admiration that this was even possible. It could be said this form of self-assessment is valuable but is prone to stroking our own egos, consequently limiting the value of evaluation; however, there is scope for more honesty and intimacy in this exchange.

Email supervision is incredibly valuable for self-assessment. Having the space to write and write and write some more, then to delete the surplus in order to write again, is cathartic. The helicopter view allows all aspects of the sessions to be examined honestly and critically. The reflective process allows noticing of what went well for the online supervisee, what will benefit the client and what didn't go so well. Making time to write also allows acknowledgement what could have been differently. Not totally focussing on the less than good but also acknowledging what has gone well, what might be useful with another supervisee and what might be expanded on in future are all important. Personally, the response I receive from my consultant is devoured as I read my words afresh and notice where my internal supervisor has assisted me or would benefit from more research, reading or requires access to continual personal development (CPD).

In formalising the process of evaluation creatively in my own work, an ever-changing formal review was constructed. The original is password protected and on this occasion there is access directly from https://fs9.formsite.com/susson/form6/index.html if it would be useful to see an example.

The form itself is composed and held in a cloud. The web site is a recommendation of an ACTO member; however, there are many similar free and paid for websites. In this case the free option continues to be secure and allows the supervisor to model the importance of sharing information securely when online. The disinhibition effect could impact in completing the form in that the supervisee may be more brutally honest than in a face-to-face session; however, for growth professionally, online supervisors can ideally welcome and hold this. The supervisory relationship is often long term, exceeding the length of non-psychoanalytic related relationships constructed with clients and will hopefully be more able to weather any storm.

Constructing the questions was a task not without challenges. Carrying out an online review to clarify expectations is preferably short in my view. Counsellors and supervisors are all busy and all prioritise what they will do at any time. Making the evaluation short enough so that the online supervisee would consider doing it immediately they opened it, but long enough to have value, is challenging. This has meant that there have been several incarnations of the document as responses and feedback have been received. There is space to elaborate and use their own words and also the option to complete it during a session if that feels more appropriate. The completion and content will be the focus of the next session regardless, as an integral part of the online supervisory relationship.

The focus of the questions is on the relationship and the supervisee's needs. It's an opportunity to indicate that a facet of the FORUM relationship needs more time or the spotlight in sessions has been skewed towards weaknesses rather than strengths, touching on personal counselling rather than supervision, for example.

The pentagons at Figure 7.4 don't fit together in any useful way. The balance is not there and they demonstrate the opposite of the collegial relationship the online supervisee seeks and the online supervisor identifies with and aims to offer. This illustration is offered as a demonstration that whilst all facets may appear to be present, they may not be beneficial. The example is extreme; however, it evidences the need for robust and timely evaluation.

Summary

Considering the many facets to all relationships, it's little wonder the online supervision relationship is one that needs careful attention. In my view, it's vital that the supervisor both understands and endorses online therapy and has gained the very specific additional training required. What we bring is ourselves to supervision and our first point of evaluation of the relationship has therefore required us to evaluate ourselves. From that base, gaining input from supervisees both informally and formally allows for the underpinning of foundations to ensure that difficult times can be weathered.

A formal evaluation can be completed easily and safely online, and the framework is therefore laid for personal growth through conversation and sharing. Constant evaluation and reviews are necessary and in order to be robust must be placed in the diary to ensure regularity and not slip past. The online therapeutic relationship is not only possible but essential in online supervision (O'Mahony, 2015).

I'll finish with this wonderful quote by Kevin Chandler (2015). I heard him ruefully say the words myself.

When it goes well supervision is most definitely the jewel in the crown. When not so well there is learning and growth so perhaps it doesn't sparkle as brightly but it's no less a jewel.

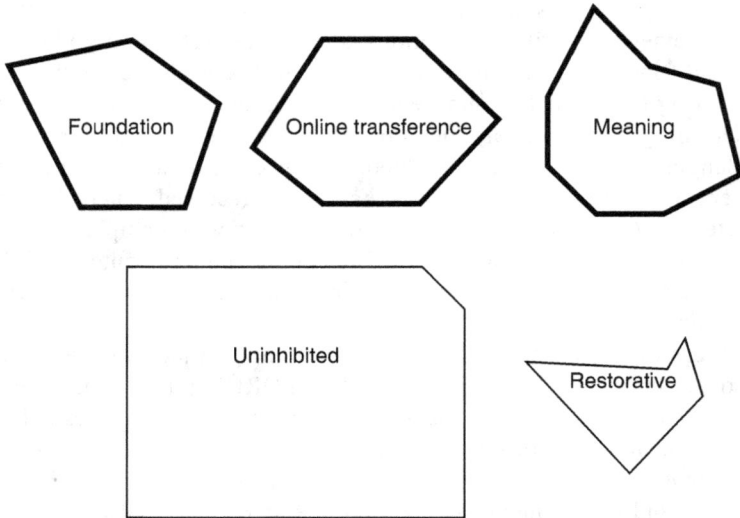

Figure 7.4 FORUM unbalanced

Note

1 Translates as:

Oh, that God would give us the very smallest of gifts
To be able to see ourselves as others see us
It would save us from many mistakes
and foolish thoughts
We would change the way we look and gesture
and to how and what we apply our time and attention.

References

BACP (2016). Frequently Asked Questions About Therapy. *BACP It's Good to Talk.* Available online at: www.itsgoodtotalk.org.uk/frequently-asked-questions/general-questions.

Beddoe, L. (2015). I wish I had known that when I started ... Becoming a supervisor: A developmental approach. Stirling University, unpublished lecture.

Beddoe, L., Davys, A. M., & Adamson, C. (2014). "Never trust anybody who says 'I don't need supervision'": Practitioners' beliefs about social worker resilience. *Practice 26(2):* 113–130.

BIBA, British Insurance Brokers' Association (2016). *A Biba Broker's Guide to Cyber Risks.* Available online at: www.biba.org.uk/current-issues/cyber/.

Bond, T. (2015). *Good Practice in Action 047: Ethical Framework for the Counselling Professions Supplementary Guidance: Working Online.* Lutterworth: BACP.

Bond, T. (2016). It really is that simple. *Therapy Today 27 (6):* 22–27.

Carroll, M. (2007). One more time: What is supervision? *Psychotherapy in Australia 13:3:* 34–30.

Chandler, K. (2015). The experience of supervision. Relationships Scotland, unpublished lecture.

Clarkson, P. (1990). A multiplicity of therapeutic relationships. *British Journal of Psychotherapy, 7(2)*: 14–163.

Counselling Tutor (2013). Petruska Clarkson – 5 relationship model explained. Available online at: www.youtube.com/watch?v=V-E1Uxw7d_g#t=11.

Feltham, C., & Dryden, W. (2006). *Developing Counsellor Supervision.* London: Sage.

Fenichel, M., Suler, J., Barak, A., Zelvin, E., Jones, G., Munro, K., Meunier, V., & Wlaker-Schmucker, W. (2001). Myths and realities of online clinical work. *Cyberpsychology and Behavior, 5(5)*: 481–497.

Hutton, D. (2012). Standing up for counsellors. *Therapy Today, 23(8)*: 28–29.

Jenner, L. (2016). The high price of empathy. *Therapy Today, 27(15)*: 28–30.

Johnston, D. (2014). *The Shadow: Our Darker Side.* Available online at: www.lessons4living.com/shadow.htm.

Kagan, N. (1974). Interpersonal process recall: Inquirer role and function. Archive.org Educational Films. Available online at: https://archive.org/details/interpersonalprocess recallinquirerroleandfunction.

Munro, K. (2002). Conflict in cyberspace: How to resolve conflict online. Available online at: http://kalimunro.com/wp/articles-info/relationships/article.

O'Mahony, C. (2015). Is an online therapeutic alliance possible? The literature to date. Onlinetrainingforcounsellors.com. Available online at: www.onlinetrainingforcounsellors.com/is-an-online-therapeutic-alliance-possible-the-literature-to-date-by-chris-omahony/.

Page, P. & Wosket, V. (1994). *Supervising the Counsellor.* London: Routledge.

Stokes, A. & Wilson, J. (2015). But I only use a bit of Skype for supervision. Onlinevents.co.uk. Available online at: www.onlinevents.co.uk/but-i-only-use-a-bit-of-skype-for-supervision-anne-stokes/.

Suler, J. (2004a). The online disinhibition effect. *Cyberpsychology and Behavior, 7*: 3.

Suler, J. (2004b). It's all in my head (solipsistic introjection). The psychology of cyberspace. Available online at: http://users.rider.edu/~suler/psycyber/disinhibit.html#anonymity.

UK Council for Psychotherapy (2012.) *Supervision Policy.* London: UKCP.

University of Sheffield Centre for Psychological Services Research. (2016). Possible difficulties within clinical supervision. Available online at: www.supportingsafetherapy.org/therapists/support-structures/possible-difficulties-within-clinical-supervision.

Yalom, I. (2002). *The Gift of Therapy: An Open Letter to a New Generation of Therapists and their Patients: Reflections on Being a Therapist.* London: Plaktus.

Yonan, J., Bardick, A., & Willment, J. H. (2011). Ethical decision making, therapeutic boundaries, and communicating using online technology and cellular phones. *Canadian Journal of Counselling and Psychotherapy, 45(4)*: 307–326.

Chapter 8

Reflective practice in online supervision

Gill Jones

Just as in face-to-face practice, online counsellors need a safe, confidential space to explore and reflect on their client work. Page and Wosket's (1994) third stage in their model of supervision is "space" and it is this reflective space that is the subject of this chapter. It is in this space that both supervisor and counsellor can explore an issue that has arisen in the counsellor's work. It is also the place without pressure and expectation where the supervisor, like Marshall's (2016) midwife, is "waiting without hope" as the session unfolds.

Just as a counsellor may choose a supervisor from the same theoretical background as themselves in order to feel truly understood, an online practitioner may choose a supervisor who works online themselves. Their mutual experience and understanding of the medium enables the counsellor to feel their experience has been truly understood. Bryant-Jeffries (2005, in Wilkinson 2015, p. 34) provides a useful definition of supervision.

> Supervision offers the opportunity to acknowledge difficulties and weaknesses, and to celebrate and value strengths and achievements. It is a place in which the supervisee can honestly and openly ask questions of his or her practice and abilities, and process what emerges, or has emerged, into awareness.

In my work as an online supervisor I believe the counsellor is the expert on their clients; my task is to create the safe space for them to step back and look at what's happening. I help them fill gaps in their knowledge and support them as they explore issues that might be hindering the work. The examples I have used here are all fictitious to avoid accidentally identifying a client who may not be aware of this book and to preserve the anonymity of all the counsellors who have worked with me as their supervisor. The examples are based on supervisory issues that crop up on a regular basis in my practice.

As there are different forms of online supervision, this chapter brings examples from all the forms I have experienced. They divide into synchronous and asynchronous supervision and within those categories there are examples from individual and group sessions. Detailed descriptions of these online supervision platforms are given elsewhere in this book; my examples demonstrate how online supervision encourages reflective practice and give a flavour of different platform styles. Although every example is written down, some sessions are spoken, using a microphone and webcam and I hope the distinctions between these and the written forms of supervision are clear. There is a brief note about each form of supervision at the beginning of the sub sections and where I have used "notes" to clarify something, it is clearly separated from the main text. In all examples, the supervisor is myself. Throughout this chapter I refer to supervisees as counsellors in the interests of clarity and simplicity (and to prevent my spell checker changing supervisees into supervises!).

Synchronous supervision and reflective practice

Supervision by webcam

Kudiyarova, in Scharff (2011), considers the difference between working face-to-face and by Skype (the most popular webcam platform) to be the difference between breast feeding a baby and bottle feeding it. The main elements of the relationship between mother and baby are the same, the difference lies in the mechanics of satisfying the baby's hunger. Other differences which also need to be borne in mind include: participants are not sitting in the same room; their view of the other person is restricted to head and shoulders; they are not making direct eye contact (most people look at the screen rather than directly at the camera); they may be using a headset to talk (more confidential when they are not in a totally private space) and the picture/sound quality can distort, pixelate (fragment) or cut off at any moment. This seemingly precarious arrangement can provoke anxiety. It needs a level of technical knowledge to handle such things as loss of sound or picture, and explicit contracting for such emergencies is essential. In this and all the synchronous examples which follow, both supervisor and counsellor have an agreed procedure for dealing with technology emergencies.

1. Jenny reflects on feeling anxious during a session with her client (Hal). Transcript from webcam supervision of a face-to-face counselling session.

This mix of supervision platforms typically happens when either the supervisor or the counsellor has changed their location either permanently or temporarily or when the counsellor finds 'local' face-to-face supervision necessitates a long journey.

Jenny has been talking about feeling anxious during her session with Hal.

Jenny: And that's it... I suddenly felt breathless whilst Hal was talking about his ex... it subsided after a few minutes. I've had panic attacks in the past so I notice my breathing but I'm not sure why I suddenly had a few panic breaths during the session – it doesn't make sense. I wasn't at all anxious before the session. It just came out of nowhere. Do you think I was feeling something in Hal that was going on underneath the surface? If so, what can I do with it?

Gill: Sounds possible, doesn't it? I'm assuming you know yourself well enough to rule out something else that might have happened to you in the hours before the session. So, let's explore this to see whether you might take it further with him. What had you and Hal been talking about just before he mentioned his ex?

Jenny: Let me think back… it was quite early in the session. He came in and sat down and I waited for him to begin and he began by saying, "it's been quite a week" (he often says that) and talked about his work; then he mentioned going out of his office for a smoke and seeing her on the other side of the road.

Gill: OK let me say that back to you – see if it helps. You began your session with Hal coming into the counselling room and sitting down. You sat waiting for him to begin and he started with "it's been quite a week". Were there any anxious feelings inside you by this point?

Jenny: No, I felt quite normal – listening and ready.

Gill: Then what?

Jenny: He talked about his work and going outside where he had the chance meeting with his ex-girlfriend and I noticed my breathing had become anxious. He said something like "funny thing, I met my ex last week – quite by chance when I left my desk for a fag" and he shifted his chair a bit further back as he was saying this. It was then I noticed my extra breaths – it was as though he wanted to get further away from me.

Gill: What do you think was happening to Hal at that point?

Jenny: I think he was uncomfortable in the room.

Gill: Something was disturbing him and you noticed it because he shifted his chair – is that right?

Jenny: Yes, I thought he was uncomfortable when he shifted his chair and my breathing was shallower than normal. If he was anxious, I was picking it up, I wonder if talking about his ex-girlfriend had made him anxious and he didn't want to go there or something else had come into his mind – perhaps to do with work?

Gill: Could you clarify that with him?

Jenny: I'd really like to if I could. Just not sure how.

Gill: Could you share your anxious feeling with him next session? Perhaps it will open up a discussion.

Jenny: Mmm – not sure. It might seem like I was leading the session and I don't usually do that.

Gill: Can you put it so that he has a choice about whether to take the discussion further or not?

Jenny: OK… let me think… I could say something like "I'm not sure if this is useful but last session I thought you were a bit anxious when you talked about meeting your ex. Would you like to explore this?"

Gill: Sounds good to me – leave him to choose. If you wait, you may find an opportunity arises naturally in a session rather than beginning with it if that feels awkward. I'd like to hear how things develop if you do use it in a session.

Supervision by IRC

This style of supervision is useful for a counsellor who is working in text chat sessions with their clients (mirroring how the counselling takes place). You will see from this dialogue that each person inputs their message more or less as they reach the end of the typing line even when they haven't finished their sentence. This keeps the words flowing and the dialogue develops a syntax and rhythm of its own. (Jones & Stokes, 2009) The convention Lisa and I have adopted is that ".." (two dots) means there is more to come from the writer. This example shows supervision providing the right space for honest reflection (Bailey, 2012 p. 30).

2. Lisa (counsellor) reflects on a practical issue with her client, Pammy.

Lisa: gotta a problem with Pammy – she paid me OK for two sessions ..

Lisa: then cancelled the third at the last minute ..

Lisa: now wants to book another session and says she can't afford to pay ..

Lisa: until her salary comes into her account ..

Lisa: I've texted it's OK to book a session once she's got the money ..

Lisa: and reminded her of my contract – pay in advance ..

Lisa: she's texted back saying she really needs a session next week ..

Lisa: says she could well have some money in account by then ..

Lisa: I don't know if I should hold the session if she hasn't paid.

Gill: Hmm that's tricky ..

Gill: Am I right in thinking she not only needs to pay you for next session ..

Gill: but also for late cancelled session as well?

Lisa: : ([keystroke equivalent of a sad face]

Gill: Have you invoiced her for the late cancellation?

Lisa: yes – she texted to say she'd pay as soon as she could.

Gill: Do you believe she will?

Lisa: I don't think she's trying to avoid paying – it's a money problem, is all.

Gill: How can you ensure you have been paid before next session begins?

Lisa: guess I could text her and explain ..

Lisa: I do have to run a business and unless the money is in my account ..

Lisa: before the start time, I'm sorry, but the session won't go ahead ..

Lisa: sounds a bit strict.

Gill: Strict? Interesting word you've used there – thinking ..

Gill: Is this also something about how you feel taking money from clients?

Lisa:	could be ....guess I feel bad about it ..
Lisa:	it's difficult charging someone who's already feeling bad ..
[pause]	
Lisa:	well that's how I feel :(
Gill:	Can I ask – did you have personal therapy in your training?
Lisa:	yep – 30 sessions spread over a year
Gill:	How did you feel about paying your therapist?
Lisa:	difficult to find the money sometimes but I never cancelled
Gill:	Sounds like you had to prioritise?
Lisa:	certainly did.
Gill:	Perhaps Pammy isn't prioritising her counselling ..
Gill:	to keep back enough money ..
Gill:	to pay for it?
Lisa:	hmm hadn't thought of that ..
Lisa:	you could be right and if we do hold our session ..
Lisa:	that may be something to explore with her ..
Lisa:	I'll send that text right after we finish here ..
Lisa:	I feel better for having talked about it. Thanks :).

Reflective supervision online can explore a gap in the counsellor's knowledge. The following example illustrates how this might be managed in a text chat supervision session.

3. Sue's online text chat client (Trish) brings an issue that is outside her current level of competence.

Sue:	My client Trish – I mentioned her last month ..
Sue:	she's been doing some writing tasks with me during our sessions ..
Sue:	she feels angry a lot of the time and doesn't know why.
Gill:	Yes, I remember her
Sue:	Well last week's session she said ..
Sue:	she'd been thinking some more about an exercise we'd done in our session ...
Sue:	I'd asked her to imagine life 5 years on, where she was living, who she was with, that sort of thing ..
Sue:	at the session she said she could see herself living in a house ..
Sue:	with someone else but she couldn't see who it was ..
Sue:	I didn't press her for more information because ..
Sue:	clients often develop their images outside the session and report back ..
Sue:	well she'd thought some more about it and she realised the other person was a girl ..
Sue:	and she now thinks she might be gay ..

Sue: thing is, I don't feel competent to help her ..

Sue: we only touched on sexual orientation in our training.

Gill: I'm checking here – she thinks she's gay ..

Gill: but she's not sure?

Sue: No, she's not sure ..

Sue: and I don't know whether I should refer her to someone who's got experience of this ..

Sue: my training course only mentioned it in passing.

Gill: Does Trish know how you feel about her disclosure?

Sue: No, I didn't said anything, I stayed with her "not sure" feeling and we acknowledged that ..

Sue: then she talked about a row she'd had at work and we looked at that ..

Sue: I let her lead the session and she didn't return to the gay issue again ..

Sue: I thought I should discuss it with you and see what I should do for the best.

Gill: Sounds like you did the right thing in the session – letting her bring it back if she chose to ..

Gill: What worries you about working with Trish who's now thinking she might be gay?

Sue: I'm worried I might say something judgemental without meaning to ..

Sue: or I might jump to the wrong conclusion ..

Sue: I'm worried I could put my foot in it without meaning to.

Gill: What options can you see for Trish?

Sue: Well – I could refer her to a gay therapist ..

Sue: Or I could continue working with her myself ..

Sue: and do some research on issues like coming out ..

Sue: read a book about it and continue working with her ..

Sue: But I'm not sure if that's the best thing for her.

Gill: Let's look at this from Trish's point of view ..

Gill: What would she choose?

Sue: I don't think she'd want to work with anyone else right now..

Sue: But this is just my feeling.

Gill: Have you thought about discussing this with her..

Gill: Seems to me what could disrupt your relationship most..

Gill: will be holding a secret ..

Gill: What about being open with Trish?

Sue: Hmm – thinking here – it could be useful ..

Sue: Trish could decide for herself ..

Sue: Yes, I think I'll lead the way with this next week. If she chooses to move to someone else we can discuss how to make an ending or perhaps take a break whilst she sees ..

Sue: someone else about her sexual orientation?

Gill: Or she could stay with you to look at her anger and then move to someone else ..

Gill: Let me know how it goes whatever she decides.

Sue: Will do. Thanks.

Online synchronous group supervision using webcam and text chat

Using these platforms can be a productive way of reflecting when the counselling is using a different online platform from the supervision. This online group has been meeting regularly for one and a half hour sessions monthly and know each other's work. All the counsellors have some online clients and use group supervision to discuss them. Each group member works in a different part of the UK and they meet up on Skype. In supervision, they share their ideas and perspectives and sometimes, as here, use role-play as a creative way of exploring an issue further (Churchill, 2013).

4. Ros, Lis, Faith (counsellors); Pat (client)

Gill: Now we're all checked in, who'd like to begin this session?

Lis: I'd like to, if that's Ok with everyone? An odd thing happened in my last text session with Pat a couple of weeks ago and I want to look at it.

Ros: Sounds interesting

Faith: Fine by me

Gill: Go ahead, Lis. We're listening

Lis: Well my client, Pat, was going on about her mother again and I began to feel angry – so I decided to share my feeling with her. Pat appeared to have finished what she was saying and I said Pat, I'm not sure if this is useful but as you were talking just now, I was feeling angry. Do you have any thoughts about that? Pat was silent for a bit then she changed the subject completely and went on about her work and how she felt over-worked but OK as she knew she could manage it. I didn't know what to do.

Faith: That sounds odd – do you think she noticed your input?

Lis: That's the problem, I don't know. I didn't know if I should return to it, or let it go.

Ros: That sounds tricky for you. What did you do?

Lis: I let it go and we discussed her work for the rest of the session. What would you guys have done? I couldn't tell if she was ignoring me deliberately or if she'd simply missed my input.

Ros: Has she talked about her mother again?

Lis: she didn't talk about her at all last week.

Gill: On balance, Lis, do you think Pat missed your input or do you think she was deliberately ignoring it?

Lis: I don't think she missed it... She's not missed anything I've written before. And she had finished what she was saying about her mother – at least I think she had. Well it sounded as though she had but perhaps I'm wrong.

Faith: Do you find Pat difficult to understand? Clients don't always say what they mean, do they?

Lis: I don't find her any more difficult than any other client – I thought we had a good relationship but ignoring what I said has me puzzled.

Gill: Lis, would it help if we role-played the exchange: you be Pat and choose one of us to be you. The others will observe and then we'll all check in with our thoughts afterwards. Would that be useful?

Lis: It might... OK let's give it a go. I'm Pat and will you be me, Faith?

Faith: I'll try.

Gill: As you work with Pat by text chat, would it help if we did this using the chat screen?

Lis: Yes that's a good idea – I'll open it up – can everyone see this?

[The group confirms that they can see the chat screen which has opened at the side of the webcam screen]

Lis: OK – here goes. I'll use .. when I haven't finished, OK Faith?

Faith: OK.

[Lis types into the chat screen]

Lis: And then she started talking about her next door neighbor ..

Lis: and how she didn't hold with her doing her vacuum cleaning ..

Lis: at all hours of the day and night. No consideration for others ..

Lis: Well by the time mother had said all that I'd stopped listening ..

Lis: she goes on and on. So I just ignore her and wait till she's finished.

[PAUSE]

Faith: Pat can I just say something here ..

Faith: it may not be helpful but as you were talking about your mother ..

Faith: I felt angry inside ..

Faith: Any thoughts?

[PAUSE]

Lis: My work was crazy last week ..

Lis: Fiona was away and I had to scoop up her work as well as *mine* ..

Lis: [speaking on webcam] I'd like to stop here if that's OK with everyone?

Gill: Of course it's OK, Lis, you're in charge. Thanks Lis and Faith, you can be yourselves again now. Can I ask you Lis, how it felt, as Pat?

Lis: As you were typing, Faith, I was feeling angry – but angry with you, not with what you were writing. That doesn't sound quite right.

Gill: Angry with your counsellor, not with the words she put on the screen? Anything else?

Lis: Yes, I felt interrupted... Faith was stopping me speaking. But it was more than that... I felt she hadn't heard me. It's difficult to put into words.

Gill: Let's see what the others felt or observed.

Faith: As the counsellor I felt I was interrupting but I did leave a pause – did you leave a pause, Lis?

Lis: Yes, I left a pause which was probably about the same length as you. I'd got a strong feeling she was waiting for me to say something next.

Faith: Yes, I felt that too. It felt as though you'd finished and you were waiting for me to write something.

Ros: I'm not sure I've got anything useful to contribute here other than I thought the way Faith phrased her input sounded caring and helpful and left the door open for Pat to use it or ignore it.

Lis: Now I've stopped to think – I'm also wondering if I touched on a feeling Pat wanted to avoid? And she could have felt angry with me for identifying it.

Faith: Sounds likely to me – your feeling may have been accurate but Pat didn't want to look at it and perhaps she was also angry that you'd noticed. I've had clients like that. Anger is something they fear exploring.

Lis: Yes – thinking about that roleplay again, I was feeling angry (as Pat) and I didn't like to have the feeling pointed out to me because I didn't want to look at it.

Gill: Lots of thoughts here. Can you use any of it with Pat?

Lis: That could be tricky. I don't want to confront or challenge her about avoiding the angry feeling – that would be counter-productive. I guess I'm going to listen out for another instance and then decide what to do.

Ros: You could try being the Alien from Mars and asking her in a spirit of curiosity if she's avoiding anger – help her have a discussion about anger and what it means.

Lis: Yes, that's a good idea – it could be useful here. Thanks Ros and thanks everyone else, this has been useful.

Gill: Please let us know how it goes.

Asynchronous supervision and reflective practice

The time-shifted nature of asynchronous supervision offers a good space for reflection, even though both counsellor and supervisor are working at different times and use an extended style of reflection in their supervision as the following examples show. As Adlington (2010) points out, when we are working with a time-lapse a question/answer format is not suitable. Questions can seem to demand an answer and the writer may not be in the same thinking space by the time they read a question in their reply. In the email examples, observations that might have been a question and answer format in synchronous supervision are here substituted with tentative reflections. In the group message board example below the use of question/answer is viable but the flow of the dialogue is freed from the need to wait for the answer before moving ideas forward.

Supervision by email

This is most suitable for counsellors who are working by email with their clients or for counsellors who have difficulty finding a supervisor they can work with in a synchronous setting (for example living abroad with poor internet connection). It has also been useful for counsellors whose supervisors are temporarily absent and who need a "sounding board" for a client issue. Here are two examples of supervision by email. Example five is a supervision session for Tom who works by email with his online clients. In this example, I suggest Tom does a short visualisation to help him. This would involve Tom reading through the visualisation and then sitting back with his eyes closed for a minute to hear the words that are in his head. The idea is adapted from Adams (1990). Example six is a regular email update from Becky which is a follow-up to a one hour/month webcam supervision session.

5. Tom (counsellor); client (Hugh)

In this example, I've placed my thoughts inside Tom's text to give a sense of dialogue. The italic text is the original email from Tom; the normal text is my reply.

Hi Tom,

I've just read your email and I'm sitting here hoping we can cast light into this dark corner. As usual I've added my thoughts inside your text [in square brackets] and I've put further thoughts at the end.

***

Hi Gill,

I have a tricky issue to bring to this supervision. I have this client, Hugh (age 75) [noticing the age difference here] *who's been emailing me for bereavement support following the death of his wife. He's an ex-pat and lives permanently abroad. He contacted me through my website because he wants someone from his own culture.* [sounds like he feels at odds with people around him] *He also said he chose me because I was a man and could understand how he felt(!)* [noticing your exclamation mark] *We've exchanged 2 emails each way and he's paid for a package of 5, so we have three more to come. My problem is I'm finding it increasingly difficult to say the "right" thing to him. I don't think we've connected at all well. He seems very quick to take offence at what I write and I feel like he's lecturing me on how to do my job.* [I'm hearing lack of connectedness, taking offence and lecturing you – a lot for you to manage] *Here's a typical example from his emails to me:*

"… to answer your question about what support system I have around me now, I'm happy to say I have plenty of people here who will sit down and listen to me going on about Cheryl. I think I'm well taken care of in that respect."

Well when I read that I thought why does he need me? [so did I] *So I wrote back saying I was pleased to hear he was using the support available to him and wondering how I could help him. He replied:*

"I look to you to help me get over my wife's death. I expect you to tell me what I can do to end this pain of being bereaved."

When I read that it felt like I was 9 years old being told off by my teacher. [Mmm, nodding my head here, it could sound like a telling off but I also notice "this pain" – wondering if there's something else as well] *I've been re-reading our emails and wondering if I've mis-judged things from the beginning. Maybe I've been empathic when really he wanted me to say "brace up, do this, this and this and you'll soon feel better" (which, of course, I wouldn't say). I'm missing something here and really need another perspective. It's de-skilling me! Help! Tom.*

***

You sound "diminished" by this client, Tom, which is so unlike you. Let's see if we can make some sort of sense out of what might be going on for Hugh – perhaps point the way to make a better connection with him. I know you use visualisation with some of your clients and I'm going to suggest you try one (I trust you not to do this if you prefer not). Maybe something useful will come out even though you only know Hugh through emails. The visualisation here is looking at Hugh's anger with you. If nothing useful comes out of it you may want to try another one with a different feeling. After you've read the visualisation through, close your eyes and see what words are in your head. Here goes.

Visualise Hugh reading your email. Imagine the setting – is he at a desk or table; or sitting in an easy chair. Is he using a laptop, tablet or mobile phone. He's opening your email and reading it. Look at his face – he's angry at what he reads. Now Hugh clicks the reply button and is typing back to you. Is he typing quickly or slowly, is he hitting the keys hard or searching for each letter.

Now keeping the image in your head sit back and close your eyes. What do you feel? Notice any words that seem to be in your head. Write them down whether you think they're relevant or not.

OK let's stop the visualisation and read through any words you jotted down. Does anything help your understanding of Hugh?

If anger doesn't work, try another feeling like sadness or perhaps fear, and try the visualisation again.

Speculating here, I wonder if Hugh's anger might mask pain which he doesn't have words for. His age suggests he grew up in an era where boys were taught to keep feelings to themselves – be strong, don't show the enemy the whites of your eyes, etc. What also strikes me, is that in spite of all the (no doubt well-intentioned) support Hugh is receiving where he lives, he still wants to discuss things with someone who is on the outside. Perhaps he's feeling "on the outside" in his local community since the death of his wife?

I hope this is useful for you. Let me know how things go – it's disheartening to work with someone you can't connect with therapeutically. Warm wishes, Gill.

6. Becky (counsellor); Edith (client). Email reflection following up webcam supervision of a webcam client

My reply to Becky's email is below.

Hi Gill, I thought I'd use this month's email to update you on the work with my rather self-contained client, Edith, who feels she's at everyone else's beck and call but is guarded about her feelings in our sessions. At our last session I noticed she was moving around in her chair. I didn't comment on it at first because the webcam view is so limited but the shifting about continued and towards the end I asked her if she was comfortable as she seemed to be moving around a lot and she said her back was bad and the chair was making it worse. Remembering what we'd said about how she may be covering up anger, I asked her if there was anything she would like to say to the chair? She said she was fed up with it, because it was so uncomfortable to sit on. I suggested that perhaps she could write a letter to the chair, listing all its failings and email it to me. I wasn't sure she'd do this but I hoped if she did, she'd let herself to be angry. A couple of days later I got a long email from her which began "Dear chair, you have always been uncomfortable and I hate sitting on you…" It sounded as though she was really letting off steam as she told the chair how it had been a dreadful chair, how she regretted ever being talked into buying it, etc. etc. It showed another side to Edith and how she feels pushed into decisions by other people. Something we can explore. She ended up saying "Sorry this is a bit long. I wrote it straight after our session. I left it on my computer for a couple of days to see if I should send it. I was upset as I wrote it but I've been feeling better since. See you next week, Yours Edith." Edith's shown me there's another Edith hiding behind the Edith who everyone turns to for help. I sent her a quick reply saying I was glad she'd sent it as it seemed to have unlocked a lot of feelings which I hoped we could talk about at our next session. Perhaps more of this sort of writing will help her explore how she can bring her inner feelings to our sessions. I'll update you at our next supervision. Becky.

Hi Becky, Thank you for the update. Well done! The task sounds just the right thing at the right moment. Getting in touch with unexpressed feelings through this type of writing is a powerful tool as Edith's just discovered. I hope she'll do more writing tasks with you. Sounds like it'll help your work with her. I look forward to an update when we next have supervision. Warm wishes, Gill.

Group asynchronous supervision

This supervision platform uses a secure, private website message board which is password protected. Members of a closed supervision group log in and leave supervision issues for each other at times which suit them. This example shows a peer group of experienced online counsellors who live and work in different countries (and time zones). They have been working together for a year by message board and have agreed a rota for taking turns to lead the group and present the topic for discussion. Although the extract below reads like a quick exchange of ideas, it could take up to week before all members of the group have added their contribution. The different inputs show support and sharing of personal experience as well as suggestion and take the issue through Proctor's (2000) normative, formative, and restorative stages effectively and concisely. It's also important that the group clarify where they are in the rota process, so their message content follows that week's lead.

Liz (UK); Mel (Canada); Maya (Ireland); Tim (US); Simon (US)

Liz: Hi everyone, I guess it's my turn to lead this week. So here goes – I've got a problem client. She's an online client who keeps silent for weeks at a time. Last time it was an 8 week gap – this time it's been 4 months! It's hard work when I do get an email from her because I need to re-read previous emails to remind myself of the issues. Anyone here got ideas about how to tackle this? <hopeful look on my face>

Mel: Hi, Liz, that's a problem – I've had it, too. I'm not sure what the best answer is about the silences, unless you want to keep prompting them that you're waiting for a reply. But I've taken to keeping a one-page summary of each client showing me when the sessions were held (or emails exchanged) and the issues covered – about a line for each. I find it helps my recall if a client returns after a long gap. Sounds like extra work when you've got the email transcript anyway but it doesn't take long and it does help when there's a gap.

Liz: Thanks for that idea, Mel, it sounds very sensible – I could give it a try.

Maya: Sounds a really clever idea, Mel, I think I'll try that, too. Not sure I've got any answers for you, Liz, but just wanted to show you I'm listening and thinking over here <smile>.

Tim: Hi Liz, thanks for bringing such a thorny issue. Email silences are a puzzle. I've had unexplained email silences from clients and often I couldn't work out why. Why does a client write one week needing your help then disappear the next week apparently not needing you any more? I used to wonder if it was my fault – perhaps I'd missed something and they'd given up on me. But when some of them checked back in, experience told me this couldn't be true all of the time. What surprises me with these client silences is that when a client comes back it's as if they've kept me in their heads all the time. They pick up where they left off. That shows me I've been an "OK" counsellor at some level <wink>. When it happens now I respect their silence and assume they have reasons for not wanting to continue. But I agree it can be a problem if the gap's been real long and they email again.

Liz: Tim that's happened to me, too – they come back and carry on it's as though there's been no gap at all. Interesting you aren't tempted to write to see if they're all right. I attach "read receipts" (an automatic reply to the sender when the email is delivered) and they nearly always send those back, then disappear after reading my email. Guess it's something I've said that's the problem <worried>. Wish I could find out.

Tim: Liz, I figured plenty of reasons why a client didn't continue – technology breakdown, life event, change of work/home, sickness. Also, you could have given them exactly the hope and resources they wanted, to move on without you! <grin>. If they remember you again – and think they need some more – they get back to you. Sure, it's possible you've written something that may have sent them away but that's only one of many possibles. We have to tolerate uncertainty and silence online and not let our feelings interfere with the work if the client returns.

Simon: Hi Liz. I'm wondering – could you contract with them that if they're silent you'll respond to their silence – remind them you're still there? Also, I know some online therapists diarise their email clients along with their in-person ones and tell them when they are available to work on their email. Don't know if that works because I don't do it myself. I prefer them to contact me when they're ready and I reply within seventy-two hours. Because I don't expect to hear from them after a particular time, guess I'm not disappointed when I don't hear <smile>.

Liz: Thanks Tim and Simon for your thoughts and suggestions. Good point Tim, about the possible reasons and not letting a silence interfere with further work if they return. You're right, Simon, I could write something into my contract that said I would make one further contact if a silence occurred after, say, not hearing for two weeks/one month (thinking aloud here) and if there's no reply, assume they no longer want counselling with me and close the file. I hadn't heard of putting session days/times into my diary but it sounds a good idea. I'll get thinking about how to do it. It's been very useful to think this through everyone, thanks.

Maya: Great idea, Simon – think I'll work on diarising my session times, too <smile>. Thanks for bringing this, Liz, it's helped me as well.

Mel: Wow – what a lot of learning here. I'm off to re-read my contract! Thanks Liz thanks Tim and Simon. This has been a really useful session for me.

Tim: It's good to hear that counsellors have the same online experiences as each other. Sounds like we're all taking something good from this week. Thanks Liz. Who's next on the schedule?

Simon: It's me next – I'll post something over the weekend. Thanks for bringing this, Liz – useful ideas here.

These examples give a taste of how reflective online supervision works in different settings. Like any clinical supervision, online supervision works best when both supervisor and counsellor have built a relationship of sufficient trust to allow difficult issues to be brought and explored in the reflective supervisory space. As Mearns (1990) says: "An important criterion in selecting a supervisor is that the chosen person should be one with whom the counsellor feels sufficiently at ease to explore even the most tortuous elements of self-doubt." The disinhibiting effect of working online with someone you neither see nor hear (asynchronous and text chat supervision) or someone who is not seated in the same room (webcam supervision) may permit some online counsellors to express themselves more freely than might otherwise be the case.

I have tried to show in this chapter that the monitoring functions of supervision can work online just as they do face-to-face. Bailey's (2012, p. 31) comment, "I am not at all sure we can ever prove conclusively that supervision works but a system that monitors everyone's process in the service of others feels a good enough check and balance to me" applies as much in online supervision as it does face-to-face. As long as the right space for reflection is created in online supervision, supervisors and counsellors will apply these checks and balances to their work.

References

Adams, K. (1990). *Journal to the Self.* New York: Warner Books.

Adlington, J. (2010). Rapport in Cyberspace. Therapy Today, 21(6): 16–22.

Bailey, C. (2012). Do We Need Supervision? *Therapy Today, 23(10)*: 30–31.

Bryant-Jeffries, R. (2005). *Person-Centred Counselling Supervision: Personal and Professional*. Oxford: Radcliffe Publishing Ltd. In: Wilkinson, E. (2015), Peer supervision and collaborative power. *Therapy Today*, May, 2015: 33–35.

Churchill, S. (2013). Transformational supervision. *Therapy Today, 24(6)*: 33–35.

Jones, G. & Stokes, A. (2009). *Online Counselling: A Handbook for Practitioners*. Basingstoke: Macmillan.

Kudiyarova, A. (2011). Psychoanalysis using skype. In: J. S. Scharff (Ed.), *Psychoanalysis Online: Mental Health and Teletherapy Training*. London: Karnac.

Marshall, N. (2016). Supervision with soul. *BACP Private Practice*, Summer: 15–16.

Mearns, D. (1990). The counsellor's experience of failure. In: D. Mearns & W. Dryden (Eds.), *Experiences of Counselling in Action*. London: Sage.

Page, S. & Wosket, V. (1994). *Supervising the Counsellor: A Cyclical Model*. London: Routledge.

Proctor, B. (2000). *Group Supervision: A Guide to Creative Practice*. London: Sage.

Chapter 9

Let's play: the improvisation of possibility in online supervision

Sally Evans

My model of online supervision isn't a new piece of theory but a tweak of a face-to-face model adapted from the work of Helena Hargaden (2016) in her book, *The Art of Relational Supervision: Clinical Implications of the use of Self in Group Supervision.*

What intrigued me about her work were the words "relational" and "self" and how they could be thought of when you provide supervision remotely via technology.

Firstly, though, what does Hargaden mean by "relational" and "self". For her, relational is at its most basic and simple level, is "how we meet each other and don't meet each other and how we meet ourselves" (p. 5). It is a philosophy which knows no theoretical boundaries so providing a framework for all clinicians regardless of theoretical perspectives. For Hargaden, it is not theory or at least not the rigid application of theory that helps people but "our personal relational abilities for emotional engagement, discernment, nuanced attunement and most of all our integrity that will inform how we work with people" (p. 1). Online or offline, it's all the same; supervision is "a relationship about a relationship about other relationships" (Fiscalini, quoted in Boyd & Shadbolt 2011, p. 280) and it's the quality of the relationship, not how you conduct it, that carries significance.

Hargaden argues that relatedness is unconscious and therefore not open to cognitive questioning so if we are to understand our supervisees and consequently support our supervisees to understand their clients, then another less content or questioning based method needs to be applied. And it is here where I believe her thinking can be clearly applied to working via technology. Because for Hargaden, it is through the interpretation of transference and counter transference which, as anybody who works online knows, are alive and well and in some instances heightened by the use of technology.

Online working allows us to have "space that is filled with a wide array of meaning and purposes", (Suler, 1998) into which unconscious processes can emerge and flourish. It is this exploration and "thoughtful disclosure and collaborative dialogue" (Hargaden, 2007) of both my inner world and the inner world of my supervisees and how they are effected, impacted upon, and heightened by that adds depth and meaning to the supervisory relationship; "working online with issues of transference and counter transference is very positive" (Weitz, 2014 p. 164).

> Transference and counter transference phenomena feature powerfully with online interactions…without the other clues (body language, etc.) that exist in F2F meeting, there is more need and, indeed, more freedom to *describe* inner responses and to request information from the other about the same. (Dunn, 2014, p. 82)

This freedom to *describe* as illustrated by Dunn fits perfectly to what Hargaden subsequently says – that relational supervision is "based on the premise that play, use of imagination, intuition, and improvisation" (Hargaden, 2016, p. 1) informs and enhances clinical supervision. It is my belief that all these elements are not only possible, achievable but gloriously present when working in cyberspace via technology. The blank screen anybody?

For example: as I read the written words on my computer screen, I often find myself momentarily staring out of the window. Is this disengagement, disinterest or an active use of dreaming? I am not suggesting we disengage with our supervisees when working remotely but simply suggesting that we can use the space we have by virtue of the distance in a creative, playful way. I have started keeping a notepad by my computer. I use it to make notes but I also doodle, I draw, I free flow and free associate with my pen and I contract with my supervisees to do the same.

Jane attends clinical supervision via synchronous text and we have a contract to work in this exploratory and creative way. In between typing and talking we both draw. We then describe to each other our "drawings" and note how similar or different they are to one another, sometimes they are and sometimes not. We also note how we feel during this process as it allows our intuitive self to emerge. This process of sharing our individual and co-created unconscious allows us to move away from a content led discussion and into a world where nothing is out of the realms of possibility. We play with possibility, not concrete facts and in doing so uncover the client in a new and exciting way.

Part of this co-experienced inner exploration also includes finding the other. Bollas states that "in order to find the patient we must look for him within ourselves" (1987, p. 202). While he was referring to a therapeutic relationship, I also then tweak this to think and apply it to the online supervisory relationship. How do I find my supervisee within me? And what do I do with "them" once I do?

I have started to see technology as a lens or conduit. A lens through which I "see" my supervisee and consequently "see" their client. Gilbert and Evans describe supervision as the "multiplicity of relationships involved in the process" (2000, p. 7). As an online supervisor, I am engaged in multiple relationships – with my supervisee, their client, with myself and with technology.

Technology as the lens allows me to observe the parallel process where the talked about relationship between myself and my supervisee becomes the "observable phenomenon" (Page & Wosket, 1994, p. 8). My supervisees find their client within our relationship but also within themselves.

> Michael is an experienced children and young peoples' online counsellor who often struggles in his supervision as to "where to start". When he does start, he either says he doesn't have "stuff" to bring to supervision or that "things" with his young clients' are going well. I find myself drawing a straight line with boxes at the opposite ends. One box is entitled "stuff" while the other is entitled "well". Out of each box, I draw another box but bigger, then smaller, then another box till I have collection of haphazard boxes of various sizes covering the page. While I'm doing so, I describe what I am doing to Michael and ask for his reaction. At first, he is startled then talks about "being boxed in" with regards his client work. He talks at length as to what "boxed in" means and feels like. Slowly he connects with Jason who now lives in residential care after a series of foster care breakdowns. Jason and his belongings have been packaged in boxes.

Technology binds all these multiple relationships together. It provides the crafted vehicle through which we can access or see not only our own subjectivity and the subjectivity of our supervisees, but these subjective explorations all take place in the space called cyber-space. Sills in her introduction to Hargaden (2016) suggests that Hargaden's relational model to clinical supervision creates a "third", a "symbolic space in which the unconscious processing [...] find resonance in each other; mind is brought to bear on inchoate experience; and nonverbal, non-conscious, and unsymbolised material can be given new meaning. This space becomes the powerful heart (Sills, 2016, pp. ix–x). This sounds remarkably like cyber-space; technology has become the conduit to cyber-space or the "third", a co-creative space where play is possible, where improvisation is possible where *description* is brought to life and used in the service of our supervisees and their clients.

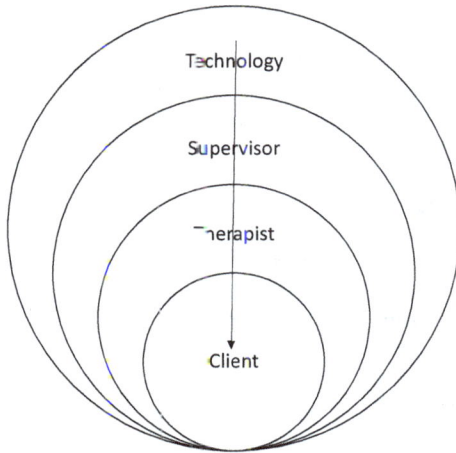

Figure 9.1 Online relationship diagram

See, my online supervisory model isn't new! While the method of engaging with supervisees may have changed, our work as clinical supervisors hasn't. The principles of ethical, effective clinical supervision remain. We simply need to think differently about the existing, creative theories we have already and to play around with them.

Reflective Question

During a supervision session, contract with your supervisee that as well as keeping written notes, you are also going to draw. Ask them if they would like to do the same. If not, you try. Draw shapes around whichever words "speak" to you. Draw shapes, doodle, let your imagination wonder and note how you feel as you do so? Do certain shapes or doodles carry more significance? Do you keep returning to certain shapes? Describe your "drawings" to your supervisee and if they have played too, get them to describe their drawings to you. As you each describe your drawings, what meaning are you making in relation to the client and the client material your supervisee brought along.

References

Bollas, C. (1987). *The Shadow of the Object*. New York: Columbia University Press.

Boyd, S. & Shadbolt, C. (2011). Reflections on a theme of relational supervision. In: H. Fowlie, & C. Sills (Eds.), *Relational Transactional Analysis, Principles in Practice*. London: Karnac, pp. 279–286.

Dunn, K. (2014). The therapeutic alliance. In: P. Weitz (Ed.), *Psychotherapy 2.0: Where Psychotherapy and Technology Meet* (pp. 77–88). London: Karnac.

Hargaden, H. & Sills, C. (2007). *T. A.: A Relational Perspective*. Bungay: Routledge

Hargaden, H. (Ed.) (2016). *The Art of Relational Supervision*. London: Routledge.

Gilbert, M. C. & Evans, K. (2000). *Psychotherapy Supervision: An Integrated Relational Approach to Psychotherapy Supervision*. Buckingham: Open University Press.

Page, S. & Woskett, V. (1994). *Supervising the Counsellor: A Cyclical Model*. London: Routledge.

Sills, C. (2016). Foreword. In: H. Hargaden (Ed.), *The Art of Relational Supervision*. London: Routledge.

Suler, J. (1998). Mom, dad, computer (transference Reactions to computer). In: *The Psychology of Cyberspace*. Available online at: http://users.rider.edu/~suler/psycyber/comptransf.html.

Weitz, P. (2014). Establishing an online practice. In: P. Weitz (Ed.), *Psychotherapy 2.0: Where Psychotherapy and Technology Meet*. London: Karnac, pp. 147–189.

Part II

Issues in online supervision

Chapter 10

Legal and ethical issues in online supervision

Kirstie Adamson

You may be a supervisor of many years of experience and you may be new to the role, whatever your position, your supervisees will look to you to support them in working with complex and difficult legal and ethical online issues.

To some extent of course the same legal and ethical issues that arise in face-to-face supervision will also arise in online supervision but there will be some additional areas to consider in online supervision. It feels important to cover these but spend more time on those which are particular to online supervision. I have included some areas of the law which I believe may arise more regularly in online supervision than face-to-face but are less well known. For a fuller exploration for legal issues I would recommend *Counselling, Psychotherapy and the Law* by Peter Jenkins (2007). The examples I have used refer to email and text supervision and counselling but of course everything applies equally to all forms of online provision.

Which Legal Jurisdiction

One of the main differences to face-to-face supervision is that when working face-to-face, the law governing the work is normally defined by where the work takes place. In online work, the participants may be in different locations and bound by different laws. In this chapter, I will be referring to the legal position in the UK.

What law is the supervision governed by? The contract can state clearly that the work is bound by the law of the supervisor's country. This is not absolute, in that any breach of contract can still be considered according to the laws of the supervisee. If there is no written contract between supervisor and supervisee then there is huge uncertainty as to which legal framework prevails. It is then more likely to be according to the law of the country of the supervisee. Different countries have different expectations of the responsibilities of a supervisor and have different laws as to the necessary qualifications necessary to practice as a supervisor. In some parts of USA, offering services without the necessary qualifications or licences can be a criminal offence (*Good Practice in Action 047: EFfCP Supplementary Guidance: Working Online BACP*, p 10).

However even in the UK I would suggest that the responsibility of the supervisor changes depending on the experience of the supervisee and the context in which supervision is being provided. If the supervisee is a trainee and not yet qualified then the supervisor will have greater responsibility. If the supervisor is being paid by the agency where the supervisee works, then the supervisor will have some responsibility towards the agency. How much depends upon the contract between the supervisor and supervisee and the agency and also the level of experience of the supervisee.

Contracts

The same requirements necessary for providing online counselling are necessary in online supervision. I see supervision whether online or face-to-face as a model for the supervisee. If a contract and clarity is necessary between counsellor and client then it is also necessary between supervisor and supervisee.

Supervision is a contract between supervisee and supervisor whether written or oral. British Association for Counsellors and Psychotherapists (BACP) recommend that this contractual relationship is reviewed not less than annually with reference to the *BACP Ethical Framework* (2016). This is going to be even more important in online supervision because things can be misunderstood.

Peter was a supervisor and had a lot of experience of working online. Sam had a small online counselling practice in a university and was looking for an online supervisor. He attended a workshop that Peter provided which impressed him. Sam liked the way Peter spoke about his client. Sam was even more pleased when he heard that Peter also worked in a university and seemed to meet all Sam's needs. They set up a contract to work together. Sam had a sense of something lacking in how Peter responded to his clients and to his work. Peter was unclear what he was doing that was not meeting Sam's needs. Sam put his ambivalence aside because he could not find any justification for it and the supervision was good enough. About a year into their supervisory relationship, it emerged that Peter worked in a university training others to become counsellors rather than counselling clients. He had assumed Sam knew this because he felt it was clear on his email endings. The client whom he had talked about in the workshop was an old client. In fact, Sam had not known this at all and had assumed he was seeing clients currently. Finding this out was a great for Sam, despite the shock, because it made sense of his feeling of not being met.

Who was responsible for this? Their contract had been set up on a misunderstanding which was not intentional on either side. What could have been done to ensure this did not happen? Could this have happened equally in face-to-face supervision as in online supervision?

If there is a written contract between supervisee and supervisor it is likely that this contract would include the qualifications of the supervisor but not necessarily the area of current work. Should the supervisee have asked or should the supervisor have made it clear?

My sense is that this was the responsibility of both practitioners. Whether you are a supervisor or a supervisee there is a responsibility to check out a situation and not make an assumption.

As you read this how many of you have a contract between you and your supervisor or supervisee for any of your work?

It can be called a contract or agreement. A contract is a legal agreement between two adults which both parties sign. It clarifies the service for which the payment is required and any conditions to this. Contracts are becoming more the norm between counsellor and client but are still relatively uncommon between supervisor and supervisee. Without a contract there can be assumptions and guesses which may be wrong and it is when things are unclear that problems can arise. This happens even more easily online.

If Peter and Sam had had a contract between them maybe things would have been clearer?

But this is based on a real situation and Peter and Sam did have a contract between them which specified the work. But neither asked the right questions to have all the information. It can be more challenging to ask these questions online as they can appear intrusive or a long list or even more dangerously, assumed which is likely what happened between Peter and Sam. In face-to-face supervision, it may be that more time is spent in establishing the relationship and checking out any questions and concerns, this still needs to happen online as well.

Ethical guidelines and supplementary guidance working online

The BACP Ethical Framework is binding on all those working within BACP guidelines whatever the therapeutic orientation or format used (s20 *Best Practice BACP*). The UK Council for Psychotherapy (UKCP) *Ethical Principles and Code of Professional Conduct* (2009) are binding on those within UKCP and there are independent bodies which other therapists subscribe to. What is important is that both supervisor and supervisee uphold the guidelines of their organisation. These are just as applicable to online work as to face-to-face work. And indeed, any work at a distance is considered to be working online.

How many face-to-face supervisors consider their emails to their counsellors to be online supervision?

How many face-to-face counsellors consider their emails to clients including arranging appointments to be working online?

Working online is wide and may be used slightly by many more people than realise it. I would therefore argue that the *Supplementary Guidance Working Online with BACP* is essential reading for all supervisors and supervisees.

The BACP Supplementary Guidance specifies that:

1. "All practitioners should be sufficiently competent in use of technology... to be able to provide reliable and adequate services to clients and colleagues" (p. 5).
2. Competence includes having an alternative method of getting in contact if your first method of contact fails and using the most reliable and most secure method of contact.
3. "It is considered good practice to receive at least some supervision online through similar technology to that used for working with clients" (p. 5).
4. Maintaining the most secure and confidential service is essential. This may change as the online world changes and so practitioners need to be up to date with this. This includes:

   a) Adequate and accessible services to clients
   b) Adequate security for services provided
   c) Vigilance to new or ongoing threats including physical and electronic intrusion

---

You are the supervisor of Thomas who is counselling Clare. You are doing SMS texting and so are working synchronously online.

In one of your sessions Thomas mentions that his partner has just come into the room.	This could be physical intrusion in that Thomas' partner could potentially read the supervision discussion. Modelling good practice for Thomas will help him to be aware of what might arise for Clare. What if her partner were to read her counselling session? What if her partner were to come in half way through a session? What does Thomas do to ensure that he closes his end of the conversation securely so that his notes cannot be read by his partner?
Thomas reports that Clare is becoming worried about other people having read her counselling sessions. Thomas knows that Clare has some paranoid ideation. Is this part of her paranoia? He is not sure whether to dismiss it or to consider anything else.	How would you know if this is a part of paranoid ideation or based on fact? This could be electronic intrusion. It would be good practice to support Thomas in working with his client to ensure: i) Password protecting documents, including transcripts, or saving them on to the cloud. ii) Password protecting the laptop or mechanism being used. iii) Check that the Wi-Fi is protected, virus protection, and spyware, etc. iv) Encryption is used where possible.

When you check out the mechanics you realise that Thomas is not encrypting emails when he sends them to Clare. Thomas is defensive about the way he works and doesn't entertain change.	Thomas has an ethical duty to keep Clare's work as safe as possible and that would include encrypting emails. I notice that whereas many counsellors encrypt their emails to clients, fewer supervisors encrypt their emails to supervisees. What is your norm? The supervisor can look with Thomas as to what is preventing him encrypting and whether this is an issue for support. If there is still a refusal then the supervisor has the sanction of reporting to Thomas' organisation, e.g., BACP and/or to stop working with Thomas. See below for impact of General Data Protection Regulations 2016 (GDPR).
Clare has asked Thomas to friend her on Facebook and Thomas is not sure how to respond.	Ideally this would be clear in Thomas' counselling contract and in your supervision contract. How social media is dealt with needs to be absolutely clear to all clients, right from the beginning. *BACP Ethical Guidelines for Good practice* states that we will ensure that "boundaries are consistent with the aims of working together and beneficial to the client" and "reasonable care is taken to separate and maintain a distinction between our personal and professional presence on social media where this could result in harmful dual relationships with clients".

Insurance

According to *BACP Ethical Guidelines for Good Practice 19*: "We will be covered by adequate insurance when providing services directly or indirectly to the public." Simply having insurance for supervision of counselling and psychotherapy is not sufficient as it needs to include working online. It is a legal responsibility to have adequate insurance for the work that you do. How many supervisors check with their supervisees about the contracts they use, their security and their insurance? I notice it is an area that often is either not mentioned or easily dismissed in supervision. It is a supervisor's responsibility to ask the relevant questions so that the knowledge is there. It is not the responsibility of the supervisor to check that it is actually carried out. That is the responsibility of the supervisee in the UK s57 *Ethical Guidelines for Best Practice BACP*.

Confidentiality

There is a common law of confidentiality which applies to counselling whether face-to-face or online. It is assumed therefore that all our work is confidential unless specified otherwise. There are legal exceptions to this and you may want to put other exceptions to this in your contract.

The legal exceptions are:

i.   The Terrorism Act 2000 provides a duty to disclose to police any belief or suspicion of terrorism as soon as is reasonably practical. Failure to do this is a criminal offence. What is more, if this emerges after work has started then it is also an offence to "tip off" your client that you are going to report.
ii.   The Drug Trafficking Act 1994 provides a duty to disclose to the police any belief or suspicion of drug money laundering as soon as is reasonably practical. Failure to do so is a criminal offence and as above, warning your client is also a "tipping of" offence.
iii. The Road Traffic Act 1998 applies only if you have witnessed an accident and the police ask you.

These exceptions need to be clear to your supervisee and your supervisee has a responsibility to make them clear to his or her clients. If this arises in the context of your work before confirming the limits of confidentiality, then it will be too late to warn their client because of the tipping off offences. If this is in the contract at the beginning of the work, then there is no problem.

Many therapists assume that child protection is a legal exception to confidentiality and must be reported. But unless you work in a protected area such as local authority, local education authority, housing, and health authority, where you are expected to share information and support enquiries, then it is not mandatory. It may well be that your ethical stance makes you want to reserve the right to report any concern regarding child protection. In which case, this needs to be part of your contract. Disclosure should be to the Social Services Emergency Duty Team or the National Society for the Prevention of Cruelty to Children (NSPCC) (Jenkins, 2007, p. 117). There is a current move towards changing the present law and making reporting child abuse mandatory. If this goes ahead, then it could raise some complex ethical issues for therapy and supervision about the role of reporting and how it impacts.

The other big exception to confidentiality is supervision as it is technically a breach and therefore the use of supervision needs to be specified within the contract. Special thought needs to be given to this when the supervision is online. There are different schools of thought as to whether first names of clients can be given within supervision or not. In online supervision, many supervisees give sections of the actual text in order to get direct support about how to respond.

Thomas has sent you an email with some excerpts from his online work with Clare. He has not deleted the client's email address from what he has sent you.	You now have identifying information regarding the client which you would never have had if you had been doing face-to-face supervision. Addressing this with Thomas is a priority. He could delete this identifying information from further supervision requests. This is a breach under GDPR.

Contrary to popular belief, in the UK there is no legal duty to report crime. In fact, it would be a breach of client confidentiality to warn an authority of the possibility of a crime taking place or having occurred unless this is specified clearly within a written contract.

Clare has told Thomas that she believes she has AIDs but that she does not want to tell her partner Sarah despite them occasionally sharing needles for recreational drugs. Thomas wants to contact Sarah to tell her of the risk of AIDs.	If Thomas had a clause in his contract that he would breach confidentiality if there was harm to self or others then he could consider reporting his client. If not, then UK law would not support him doing this (Jenkins, 2007, p. 125). Good practice would support him bringing this issue up direct with Clare regardless of the terms of his contract to look at concerns.

Good practice would always mean that unless there was an issue under the Terrorism Act or the Drug Trafficking Act which prevented disclosure to the client, then the supervisee should first discuss any potential breach of confidentiality, where possible, with the client. This should always be an issue that is brought to supervision.

The Data Protection Act 1998 and General Data Protection Regulations 2016

In the UK, personal data has been governed by the Data Protection Act 1998 (DPA). On May 25th 2018 the General Data Protection Regulation 2016 (GDPR) comes into effect.

• Personal Information is any data which relates to an identified or identifiable natural person including racial or ethnic origin and biometric data, sexual life, political opinions, religious or similar beliefs, membership of trade union, physical or mental health, commission of offence, processing of offence

- All handwritten notes are relevant if they are kept in "relevant filing systems" e.g. when data is structured so that specific information relating to an individual can be identified.
- If any personal process notes are identifiable they become part of the client's records.

The principles of the GDPR Act are:

1. Processed fairly and lawfully and transparently.
2. Collected for specific and legitimate purposes – information given in therapy cannot be re-used for another purpose. Reprocessing for archiving is legitimate.
3. Adequate, relevant and limited to what is necessary – what do you need to record to fulfil the purpose of keeping notes?
4. Accurate and where necessary up to date – not misleading or incorrect and erased or rectified if not.
5. Not kept for longer than is necessary -how long is appropriate to keep notes after the end of the therapeutic relationship?
6. Processed so as to ensure the security of the personal data including no unauthorised or unlawful processing or accidental loss, destruction or damage with appropriate technical or organisational measures.
7. Keeping notes in a locked cabinet, keeping computer notes password protected and on a cloud.

Each person has the:

- Right to be informed of any information held on them e.g. personal data as well as any notes kept.
- Right of access to any information stored, within a month mostly without charge.
- Right to rectification if anything is inaccurate.
- Right of erasure so that items can be deleted.
- Right to restrict processing i.e. not to give a client's details to another body.
- Right to portability-clients can ask for their data and can reuse this for their own purposes.
- Right to object to what is done.
- Right not to be subject to automated decision making e.g. excluding person for race, postcode etc.

GRPR clearly has huge potential for all counselling work whether online or face-to-face but if we are compliant with DPA then it should not be difficult to comply with GDPR. At the time of writing, GDPR has not come in to force. Checking and reviewing in supervision where and how personal data is being held several times a year will support supervisees to show compliance. We will all need to hold, review the data, amend or update the data and maintain data on a regular basis. Non-compliance can incur a fine of 4% of turnover or 20 million euro. In face-to-face supervision, none or only brief notes are taken by either supervisor or supervisee, but in online supervision the whole of the supervision could be open to scrutiny. What are appropriate guidelines for keeping supervision records? Does this differ when it is online supervision? Can it be different from counselling notes? All these are valuable questions, for which there is no set rule or answer and is an individual decision. The guidance is as above "not kept for longer than is necessary". Many people hold notes are kept for three or six to seven years, not because there is a guideline for this but because three years is the limit for negligence proceedings through the courts and six years is the limit for issuing civil proceedings through the courts. Some people keep supervision notes for the same time as counselling notes whereas others keep them only until their next supervision session. Some years ago, I carried out a survey (unpublished) in Bristol of how long counselling notes were kept for and the responses went from no notes being made, to keeping notes for twenty years. GDPR means that you need to be clear why you are keeping notes, for what purpose and that your supervisee knows these notes are kept?

In online supervision the fact that the notes consist of the whole of the supervision session. This may impact on how long a supervisor decides to keep notes. Some online practitioners go to the lengths of writing separate brief notes and not keeping the actual session. This seems unnecessary to me as the client will already have the whole session. Whilst you may have your own guidelines for how long you keep your supervision notes for, your online supervision notes may be kept for far longer by your supervisee. As a supervisor, this is not your decision but the supervisee's.

Registration with the Information Commissioner's office is essential as any form of online supervision will necessitate this. You are a data controller and liable to registration if you process any personal information on your computer even if it is deleted straight away. This could be as little as an email about appointments or a text message to a client. The process is straightforward and there is an annual fee. From April 2018 this will be £55. The website for the Information Commissioner's office is www.ico.gov.uk

Request for disclosure of notes

If a request is made by a client or the courts or the police (with the client's consent) for all notes concerning a client, then any supervision records that have been kept by the supervisee may form part of the notes and will have to be disclosed by the supervisee. The notes can however be redacted. This means that comments by the supervisor that are about the client will need to be left as they concern the client, but comments about the supervisee do not concern the client and so they can have a black line drawn through them so that they cannot be read.

> *Reading this sounds as if you were upset and really felt for the client.* This feels very moving for the client.

The above italics refer to the counsellor and not the client and so can be redacted. In order to comply with the act, it is important that it is clear to those requiring notes what is being redacted. A black line through each word making it illegible is sufficient. If there is external supervision, then this is not relevant as if it was deemed essential for supervision notes to be disclosed it would be a separate data protection request to the supervisor.

The requests for notes to be disclosed are increasing and in certain agencies and organisations this is more common than others.

In relation to a request for notes by the police without the client's consent then it is possible to refuse to disclose these until an order is made by the court. An order in the civil court would be under ss 33 & 34 of the Supreme Court Act 1981 and in the criminal courts under the Police and Criminal Investigations Act 1996. In my experience, I have rarely known notes to be requested without the consent of the client. Some practitioners are still writing therapeutic notes e.g. about their feeling and opinions in an identifiable form which means they are disclosable. If an order for disclosure is made by the court then refusal to provide notes can be seen as contempt of court. Sometimes the offer of a brief report might be accepted and this avoids the need to disclose sometimes sensitive information which has no relevance to the court proceedings.

Suicidal ideation and self harm

Contrary to general opinion, just as there is no duty to report crime in the UK, so there is also no duty to prevent suicide. Under the *BACP Ethical Guidelines*, the list of values includes, "Alleviating symptoms of personal distress and suffering" and "Protecting the safety of clients" (BACP, 2016, p. 3). However, in law this does not mean that the therapist or the supervisor is responsible for preventing suicide or self-harm. In law, a person is responsible for damage to another if a duty of care can be proved. In the UK at present there is no duty of care for suicide or self-harm. This means that it is not the responsibility of a supervisor to prevent suicide in the UK but to act ethically.

Suicide is increasing and according to the World Health Organisation (2012):

- Nearly one million people kill themselves worldwide every year
- This amounts to sixteen per 100,000 people or one person every forty seconds and has increased by 60% for the last 50 years
- Suicide is the leading cause of death for those between fifteen to forty-four years old.

This means it is extremely likely that at some point every supervisor will have a supervisee with a client who has suicidal ideation. Managing suicidal ideation online can often feel much more nerve-wracking than face-to-face because of the distance in working.

It will depend on the terms of your supervisee's contract with the client as to whether or not concerns can be reported to a GP or other professional. An adult client with mental capacity, who is considering suicide, has the right to refuse disclosure to a third party. This is another example of why a clear contract is vital at the beginning. Without this clause in the contract there is no consent to disclose information and disclosure could be a breach of confidentiality and without consent. There would however be grounds to justify such a breach on the basis of working with the BACP principles of beneficence and non-maleficence.

When working at a distance with a client, your supervisees will not necessarily be able to recommend local support agencies. It becomes important therefore to be aware of national agencies and help that can be contacted online such as:

www.getselfhelp.co.uk/suicidal.htm
www.nhs.uk/Conditions/Suicide/Pages/Introduction.aspx
www.papyrus-uk.org
www.samaritans.org

Thomas brings a client, Andrew, to supervision. Andrew has been very suicidal. Thomas is nervous about "talking" about this openly with Andrew as he does not want to increase the risk of Andrew taking his life.
He is especially anxious because this is online work.

Ongoing risk assessment is essential in all therapy especially when there is suicidal ideation. Research has proved that asking direct questions does not increase the risk of suicide. Clear questions can support the client in feeling valued, listened to, and less alone.

Some agencies will not work with clients on suicidal ideation online and insist on having face-to-face sessions. What happens if a suicidal client refuses face-to-face sessions and then stops further sessions?

Providing information about resources is always valuable such as Samaritans, Mind, and other websites.

Thomas confirms that he has heard that Andrew went ahead and ended his life. He is struggling with whether he could have done more.
He has had a letter from Andrew's family asking him for disclosure of his notes as they want to understand the reason for Andrew's death.

A client is responsible for his own life and ultimately a counsellor is not responsible for a client's choices. What would you have done differently?

Confidentiality of the client remains with the client even after death. There are no rights of disclosure of the notes to family after the client's death.

Disclosures

Online work is commonly known as a form that can encourage disclosure, as Suler discussed in the "Online disinhibition effect" (2004). Therefore, disclosures of previous abuse may be more common in online work. The increase of disclosures in the public arena in recent years has also supported more victims to come forward.

It is important to be aware of the guidelines for providing therapy for victims who are involved with court proceedings – www.cps.gov.uk/publications/pretrial adult.htm.

Vulnerable witnesses may need support in order to take an issue to court. Primarily what is most important is what is in the best interests of the victim. However, there is a conflict between the needs of the victim to receive the best support to enable their recovery and also a fear of tainting the evidence by discussion in therapy. It also needs to be remembered that all therapy notes may well be requested up to the date of the trial. Best practice guidelines confirm that:

i) Some therapeutic work may prejudice the outcome and/or impact the evidence before the court.
ii) Issues that have less impact on a court case might include issues on self-esteem, "reduction of distress about the impending legal proceedings" and any emotional issue "that does not require the rehearsal of abusive events".
iii) Therapy should be stated before it begins and both therapist and witness need to be aware of the court proceedings and the Crown Prosecution Service needs to be informed.
iv) Clear records need to be kept in case disclosure is requested.

This can be incredibly difficult for both parties and it is best if the guidance is read at the time if such a case arises.

An important resource in these circumstances is a Sexual Assault Referral Centre (SARC) which is a single point of access for anyone who has been sexually assaulted. Whether or not a victim wishes to report an assault to the police a SARC can still offer support and counselling. SARCs will on request provide a special place for victims of assault to be supported, give statements, and if appropriate have a personal examination. Even if a victim does not want to report an incident immediately a SARC can take the evidence and hold it for a later date. There are now many SARCS throughout the UK and can be easily located. This does not preclude a report to police and it is up to the victim and not your supervisee or you as supervisor as to how the client proceeds.

Prevent

Prevent is a government strategy to prevent terrorism: www.gov.uk/government/publications/prevent-duty-guidance.

This was developed to increase knowledge of radicalisation and to help us all to understand what we can do and how we can support others from risk of radicalisation and from being involved. There is an explicit duty with "specified authorities" which includes schools and universities. Here is a link to some general training about Prevent: www.elearning.prevent.homeoffice.gov.uk/.

This does use examples of pupils at schools but may help anyone working with someone who appears to display signs of radicalisation. It shows how much the indications are often small and only significant when linked together. Isolation is often a significant factor which may be why this may come up in online work. But it also shows that it is important not to make assumptions and to seek adequate supervision.

Thomas' client Clare has in the past felt very supported by her partner Sarah. Recently however Sarah has been distancing herself and is talking more and more about this new group of people she has met. She won't allow any demonstration of affection between herself and Clare in public and calls Clare her flat mate. Clare has said that Sarah is talking about her mission in life and has become more right-wing. Thomas got the feeling that there was a risk of radicalisation but didn't want to ask her or probe any further. He feels that Clare will not say anything more if he was to ask	How will you support Thomas? What is your duty as a supervisor? Knowing something about the duties of Prevent will help you with this. In this case study excerpt, there is no clear evidence, which is often the case and so it is important not to make assumptions but to seek support and advice.

Living wills

Having a living will is essential for any therapy practice. What does a living will mean? It means having arrangements in place for your clients in case of you dying or suffering any incident that prevents you from contacting your clients personally and prevents you being present for your sessions. When a volcano erupted in Iceland and brought most air traffic to a complete halt I happened to be in India. At the time, I was told that it would be months before I would get back to the UK. I did manage to get back within less than a week. I would not have got back in time for any of my clients and I was very grateful for my living will. Potentially I could have done online work provided that I could have arranged sufficient security but some of the time was spent travelling back. In other situations it might be spent in hospital. It is not the responsibility of the supervisor to arrange this for the counsellor but it is the responsibility of the supervisor to raise this with their supervisee. All supervisees need to ensure that a responsible person can have access to a means of contacting all clients. It is not appropriate for this to be a family member.

Summary

I have not tried to look at all legal and ethical issues as this would be more the subject of a whole book but I have given a brief overview and looked at those which are particularly relevant to online supervision and may be least well known.

According to the *Good Practice guide of the Ethical Principles* (BACP, 2016)

"Supervision requires additional skills and knowledge" this is even more the case in online supervision. s55 and s59 of the *Ethical Framework* requires supervision to review how the framework applies and is working "regularly and not less than once a year". What this means and how it can be demonstrated is yet to be seen.

What is important is that supervision online requires additional forethought and additional knowledge so that it supports supervisees to provide the best provision for all clients

References

Bond, T. (2016). *Ethical Framework for the Counselling Professions.* Lutterworth: BACP.

Bond, T. (2015). *Good Practice in Action 047: Ethical Framework for the Counselling Professions Supplementary Guidance: Working Online.* Lutterworth: BACP.

Great Britain (1981). The Supreme Court Act 1981. London: Stationery Office.

Great Britain (1994). The Drug Trafficking Act 1994. London: Stationery Office.

Great Britain (1996). The Police and Criminal Investigations Act 1996. London: Stationery Office.

Great Britain (1998). The Data Protection Act. London: Stationery Office.

Great Britain (2000). The Terrorism Act 2000. London: Stationery Office.

Jenkins, P. (2007). *Counselling, Psychotherapy and the Law.* London: Sage.

Jones, G. & Stokes, A. (2008). *Online Counselling: A Handbook for Practitioners.* Basingstoke and New York: Palgrave Macmillan.

Suler, J. (2004). The online disinhibition effect. *CyberPsychology and Behavior,* 7: 321–326

Websites

www.cps.gov.uk/publications/pretrialadult.htm

www.elearning.prevent.homeoffice.gov.uk/

www.getselfhelp.co.uk/suicidal.htm

www.gov.uk/government/publications/prevent-duty-guidance

www.ico.gov.uk

www.nhs.uk/Conditions/Suicide/Pages/Introduction.aspx

www.papyrus-uk.org

https://www.psychotherapy.org.uk/.../UKCP-Ethical-Principles-and-Code-of-Professional-conduct

www.samaritans.org

Chapter 11

Online supervision and managing risk in an international context

Lalage Harries

Introduction

What is a feature of online supervision which is impossible to create without the online context? Working across international borders: No other means of practising supervision could make working simultaneously in different countries, without either necessarily ever being physically present in the others' context so feasible or so attractive.

This creates scenarios which would not have existed before online counselling and supervision and provokes questions our profession may not have considered: How do we manage our supervisory responsibilities across different legal and regulatory contexts? How do we even identify them? How do we manage potential conflicts between them?

What this chapter is about

In this chapter, I will explore some challenges and opportunities in supervising work across international borders, with particular emphasis on identifying and managing risk. I will explore some of the features and questions peculiar to online international supervision, using case studies to illuminate different questions. I will look at legal and regulatory constraints supervisors may need to consider, and touch on some contextual differences supervising within an organisation or individual practice may entail. Finally, I present a checklist of potential areas for consideration when planning to work with internationally based supervisees.

This grew from reflections on my experiences as online supervisor and draws on the research and learning which developed as I worked to answer the questions I posed in the introductory paragraph. The case studies presented are anonymised collations drawn from real cases.

Any supervision, let alone internationally based supervision, must raise many questions around the cultural and social context of the supervisory relationship and clinical work. This must require serious and ongoing consideration if the relationship and quality of the work are to prosper (Collins & Arthur, 2010; Crockett & Hays, 2015; Ng & Smith, 2012). However, it is not within scope of this piece of writing to attempt to engage with these huge topics in the depth they surely deserve. Whilst it is impossible to avoid discussion of context, I would warmly invite the reader to use the bibliography of this chapter for further reading sugges- tions on this rich and complex topic. The previous chapter also refers to the legal issues which may arise.

Who this chapter is for

Whilst this chapter will be of particular relevance to those working directly with supervisees based outside the UK, the issues raised are of increasing relevance to the wider online and face-to-face therapeutic community. With the "increas- ing internationalisation of the world" (Leong & Ponterotto, 2003, p. 382) we see ever greater fluidity in work and travel arrangements for counsellors and clients alike. We may find that a framework for considering international responsibilities as a supervisor may be necessary, even when you have no intention of planning to work with internationally based supervisees, as this chapter will demonstrate.

Key responsibilities in supervision

This might be a good moment to clarify what responsibilities we are discussing when we contract to work with a supervisee, international or not. How do we define the task in hand?

This summary of perspectives from some key figures in supervision theory provided by Sagganjanavanich and Black is a good start:

> [T]he supervisor aims to foster and enhance the supervisee's professional development and competence as well as to ensure the client's welfare through the monitoring of the quality of professional services. (Bernard & Goodyear, 2009; Falender & Shafranske, 2004; Watkins, 1997 in Sagganjanavanich & Black, 2009, p. 52)

Whilst we seek to assist the supervisee flourish in their work, arguably our most important supervisory responsibility is "to monitor/safeguard the interests of the client" (Despenser, 2011, p. 2) and ensure that the therapeutic support provided maintains appropriate ethical standards for all parties.

As BACP online counselling and psychotherapy guidelines remind us:

> Supervisors should be aware of the legal and professional regulations as they apply in the country, state and professional organisations of both supervisee and supervisor.... All therapeutic and supervisory practice should comply with applicable law and policy. (Anthony & Goss 2009, p. 11)

How can we ensure we provide supervision which is not just legally, but socially and culturally relevant to our supervisees' practice? Finally, what criteria can we apply to establish our potential competence to support an internationally based supervisee in their context?

Lack of published literature

On beginning initial research into this question, I was struck by the lack of literature currently available on this particular topic. I found publications on working in international settings as a face-to-face practitioner (Gray, 2015) and on international therapists' experiences working in the UK (Costa, 2014; also Georgiadou, 2015), texts on the provision of multiculturally competent supervision (Crockett & Hays, 2015; Collins & Arthur, 2010; Robinson, Bradley & Hendricks, 2000) and on working face-to-face with international supervisees (Alberta & Wood, 2009; Ng & Smith, 2012); texts on the internationalisation of the therapeutic professions (Chang, 2013; Leong & Ponterotto, 2003; Ng & Noonan, 2012; Stannard, 2013), and on online supervision within national borders (Orr, 2010; Wright & Griffiths, 2010).

Whilst I found some scholarly articles and books identifying that there were legal and regulatory considerations to be made, these were largely focused on USA perspective (Anthony, 2009; Zack, 2008). Anthony, Goss, and Nagel (2014) provide a useful starting point in considering factors involved in ethical cross border practice and *The Need for and Barriers to International Regulation* (Goss & Anthony, 2009) engages with the implications of international differences; however, this discussion is limited to a few paragraphs.

It is regrettable that there is little research and writing in this area, particularly from a supervisory standpoint, as finding an ethically and legally appropriate response to working with internationally based supervisees may be of increasing pertinence for online supervisors. The UK therapeutic community has been a relatively early adopter of online counselling with a number of well-established online training courses and practitioners.

As an English-speaking country presenting few regulatory barriers to international online practice in comparison the USA for example (see Gray, 2015), UK online supervisors may well be a first port of call for many internationally based, newly established online counsellors, seeking a more experienced online supervisor.

Case study

Cristina is an Italian counsellor, who had trained in a primarily psychodynamic model in Italy, where she lives and works. She has wide ranging experience in working in charity settings with children, refugees, and domestic abuse survivors and had recently completed an online counselling training diploma with a UK based online counselling training organisation.

Cristina is passionate about the potential of online counselling and was keen to be amongst the first to introduce it to a country where she felt it was still relatively unknown. She reported to me that as there was no online counselling training in Italy and no supervisors trained to work with online counsellors, she had sought out training and supervision from the UK. This would not have been possible for her if she did not speak English, though her first language – the one she counsels in – is Italian.

One of the clients Cristina presented in supervision was a woman in the process of an acrimonious separation from her husband, also the father of her nine-year-old son. The client had reported some stalking and verbal abuse from her husband and had been given details of the local women's refuge and a legal support team who specialised in domestic abuse cases but had chosen not to pursue this.

Whilst no outright violence had occurred, the child had been coerced by his father into spying on his mother by threatening to withdraw his affections from the child. He had also witnessed his mother's family physically prevent his mother from leaving the house during an argument where the husband had become physically threatening. Despite this, Cristina's client did not want to take any action beyond sharing this in counselling.

At this point, child protection concerns might be expected to be raised externally by a counsellor: I wanted to understand why Cristina was not considering this as an option to pursue. Cristina told me that as a counsellor in Italy working in private practice, she had fewer legal rights to break confidentiality than a counsellor in the UK. We also discussed differences in legal thresholds for child protection between the UK and Italy and Cristina's expectation that this child's experience would not hit any thresholds for intervention under Italian law.

Cristina also identified that in Italian society the family remains a dominant paradigm whose authority and sanctity is not easily challenged. These cultural thresholds, which are always at play in how a law is enacted, also needed to be factored when considering an effective and ethically sound intervention.

Whilst I respected my supervisee Cristina's work and trusted her care for her clients, I was faced with a dilemma; the only source I had for this new information about the therapeutic context in Italy was my supervisee. This felt too precarious when I took supervisory responsibility for her work and potential risks had been identified. With UK based supervisees I would consider it my responsibility to be independently informed to the best of my ability; it could not be different here though the task might be more challenging.

The research I undertook fully endorsed Cristina's perspective on her client's situation (see Bertotti, & Campanini, 2013; *Codice Penale*, 2016; Leveille &

Chamberland, 2010; Montero, Jay, Owen, & Korintus, 2014; Saulini (Ed.), 2002; Remley, Bacchini, & Krieg, 2010.). However, if this had not been the case and the issues had not been fully explored in supervision, then the overriding responsibility – client welfare – may well have suffered.

Beginning research

I asked myself what knowledge about the working practices and context of a UK based supervisee I might hope to grasp with relative speed and ease and created the following list, which formed the basis of my research and came up with the following list:

- Language
- Regulations & qualifications
- Laws
- Resources
- Shared social context

However, it should be acknowledged that none of these can be taken for granted, nor are they straightforward. UK law differs in Scotland, England. and Wales for example. The requirements of the many therapeutic regulatory bodies or the precise level of training different UK based courses offer can be labyrinthine in their complexity.

The notion that even amongst native English speakers, language will be used and understood uniformly regardless of age or location is immediately suspect. Similarly, the idea that someone based in a small town in South East England (like me) will understand the context of an online supervisee based in Ibrox, Glasgow or rural North Wales without some reflexive processing, research and internal translation would be highly misleading.

What may allow us to feel some measure of confidence in navigating these things in the UK is spending years steeped in a shared national context. A high level of contextual knowledge is necessary to understand and interpret data concerning therapeutic practice here or elsewhere.

Through each heading I asked myself what questions I needed to answer, what processes I needed to put in place to close the gap sufficiently to work effectively with an internationally based supervisee.

Language

Language is often the primary currency of therapeutic work. Walsh (2014, p. 60) asks: "Who am I as a therapist in a particular language? Who is the patient in a particular language? What is the specific language-related relationship created between us" – a question that might also be asked of the supervisory relationship.

As Walsh indicates here, and as Charura (2014) explores in an online counselling context, we are different selves expressed through different languages. If for example, your supervisee works with clients in their native language and receives supervision in a non-native language, what changes in how information is conveyed, or understood?

How sophisticated does the shared understanding of language between supervisor/supervisee need to be to:

a)   Convey complex emotional meaning from client sessions
b)   Convey accurate factual information which may be needed to assess risk

There can't be a simple answer to those questions, it will vary within each supervisory relationship. However, considering how much content can be accurately covered in a session using a second language may be important, as you may find longer is needed to provide reasonable cover of the supervisee's concerns.

It may also take longer when working with someone in a second language to establish the amount of time needed and how language use differs between written and verbal communication. When I first began supervising Cristina, we contracted after a second meeting to work primarily in a live video based platform and to add an additional half hour of asynchronous text following supervisions to confirm actions, share reflections, and catch potential language based confusion so that any misunderstandings could be swiftly identified and managed. If bringing transcript excerpts from client sessions to supervision, consideration may be given to who translates this, and whether the original text may also be examined.

If the supervisee is working somewhere where the principal language is not spoken by the supervisor, then the supervisor's capacity to conduct independent research will undoubtedly be affected by their ability to navigate the language at least at a basic level. A variety of online translation tools can assist in the research process, but some language knowledge not only speeds and improves research, but also enhances the alliance with the supervisee (see Kapasi & Melluish, 2015).

Regulations & qualifications

When first contracting with a supervisee, establishing their competency to practice – and yours to support their practice – is obviously vital. Different legal and regulatory requirements may be in place in your prospective supervisee's context which might not be immediately apparent. Speaking of online counselling, Bond reminds us that it is "good practice [...] to be familiar with legal requirements" when working internationally (Bond, 2015, p. 11). Both Bond and Anthony highlight limitations to practicing internationally: "Legal stipulations exist in pockets around the world, such as in America" (Anthony, 2015, p. 39).

You may need to ensure it would be appropriate for the supervisee to receive supervision from you, checking the terms of any registration or licencing to which they may be subject. Similarly, some counsellors will find their insurance may or may not cover them to offer any therapeutic services, including supervision, in some international territories.

Some further questions to clarify when contracting are:

o   Is the supervisee qualified to their country's standards and allowed to practice?
o   Are they in training and does that make additional requirements of them (and potentially of their supervisor)?
o   Are they insured and a member of an organisational body with a complaints procedure?
o   Is supervision a regulatory requirement and what requirements are made of it?

In some contexts, there may be little regulation of therapy and careful consideration should be given to contracting with a supervisee where there may be no clear recourse for their clients should they wish to complain or take action against the supervisee's work. If proceeding, you may need to think together about additional contracting to acknowledge and mitigate, perhaps agreeing to work to the supervisor's ethical code.

Thought might also be given to the supervisee's expectations of supervision. In some contexts, including those where supervision is a well-established and embedded profession, supervision is not a continuous requirement after training (see Wright & Griffiths, 2010, p. 692) and supervisees may see it as an ad hoc activity to be taken up as needed. This may jar with UK based supervisor expectations and thought should be given to what contractual agreement will be mutually satisfactory from an ethical and practical perspective.

As well as incorporating questions into a contract for completion by the supervisee, care should be taken to talk through these questions thoroughly and gain a full understanding of the supervisee's regulatory requirements, limitations, and expectations. This was reinforced to me when working with my Italy based supervisee:

Example

I had understood that distinctions existed between "counsellors" (which is an unregulated profession) and "psychotherapists" (which is regulated). However, other regulatory differences were less clear, such as the distinction made between those working in a "public" setting (e.g., governmental) or a "private" setting (private company, charity, independent practice, etc.).

A series of laws outline the different level of weight a declaration of concern for the welfare of a client would carry with Italian authorities, and the legal injunctions both to disclose *and to not disclose* concerns, depending on your role (counsellor/psychotherapist) and your setting (private/public) there are clear limitations to breaking confidentiality, even where risk is known to the counsellor (see *Codice Penale*, pp. 361, 362, 365, & 378).

This localised issue illustrates that we cannot take for granted how differently an idea as central to our work as confidentiality may be held in legal and regulatory practice internationally. I do not think I could have hoped to find the relevant legislation and guidance on this without clear and detailed pointers on what I should be looking for, to which only a contextually situated person (in this case, an Italian psychologist friend of a friend) could direct me.

In this instance, the power of an international network of local knowledge would be invaluable to an online supervisee. National and international online counselling organisations could play a valuable role here which I discuss further at the end of this chapter.

Laws

Safeguarding and child protection

The law is the basis on which action may or may not be taken. Nowhere is this felt more acutely than in safeguarding and child protection. In our UK-based practice, we need and expect to have a working knowledge of relevant UK laws; thus we may see the direct impact that changes in the law have on client safety.

Example

In 2015 new guidance on controlling and coercive behaviour in abusive relationships was provided as part of the Serious Crimes Act 2015.

Senior staff at a charity based counselling service reported that due to the change in the law, guidance for thresholds for external referral was changed. As a result, several cases of domestic abuse were referred to the police that would not have met safeguarding thresholds the previous year.

We also know that it is the marginal calls, sitting on the edge of safeguarding thresholds which need a most thorough understanding of law and its application, and are perhaps most in need of careful teasing out through supervision.

This is also where we are likely to see the greatest variance in whether an equivalent law exists in another country and how it is phrased. As the example above demonstrates, a slight difference in phrasing, emphasis or guidance to professionals on the execution of the law will result in different outcomes for vulnerable clients.

The disjuncture between UK Government safeguarding guidance requiring us to observe both local and UK law when working internationally (see UK Government, 2014; SAFE CIC, 2015) is clear here. If the law where the client is based is not parallel to UK law, there is at least some un-resolvability, however much we seek to fulfil our responsibilities under UK safeguarding law and our regulatory body's code of conduct (see also the previous chapter).

An understanding of the relevant laws, transparent discussion with the supervisee, your regulatory body and your own supervision of supervision may all strengthen good practice here. Similarly, a good local understanding of how the law is applied and managed is also needed to be effective as considerable variance within national borders has been observed by both national and international researchers. For further discussion of this, see Bessant (2011), Johansson (2010), and Benbenishty et al (2015).

Example

A UK online children's counselling service contracted to train counsellors in another EU country to work online, using the UK model as a template for the new European service's practice. The UK service offered counselling without parental consent to young people over eleven years old who demonstrated "Gillick competence". However, no such legal guidance existed in this new setting and it was deemed mandatory under this country's law to seek the consent of parents/guardians when counselling anyone under eighteen years old.

Careful planning and discussion through supervision of both sets of counsellors was needed to establish a new protocol for working together which satisfied the legal/regulatory and ethical needs of both the UK and international children's counselling services.

Data law

All therapists need to consider the management of sensitive data, but this becomes a more complex question when considering data which will be transferred between the UK and another country. The eighth principle of The Data Protection Act 1998 is particularly relevant to this question; it states that:

> Personal data shall not be transferred to a country or territory outside the EEA unless that country or territory ensures an adequate level of protection for the rights and freedoms of data subjects in relation to the processing of personal data. (ICO, 2012, p. 83)

Whilst there are no restrictions on the transfer of data between EEA countries, it is important to understand what laws govern data management including:

o   Consent
o   Third party access
o   Deletion of data

as legal requirements on how data is processed once it has arrived may differ within EEA countries. This may be particularly relevant if your supervisee is working in a larger organisational setting rather than private practice, where others may have access to client information.

When contracting, it is important to clarify the supervisee's expectations of data security, encryption, and client consent as well as outlining your own data security processes. Ensure you have the supervisee's explicit consent to transfer their personal data, especially if they are based in a country to which the EU commission has not given "positive finding of adequacy" (ICO, 2012, p. 84). If your supervisee is based in a country deemed to have poor data security, you may want to discuss putting in place additional steps for security and anonymisation to ensure the safety of client data.

Within supervision, it should be possible in most cases to anonymise client information so that little or no personal information is transferred internationally. Detailed guidance on anonymising data can be found via ICO website listed below. In the interests of transparency, supervisees may advise clients that their supervisor is UK based, as part of fully outlining their data management processes when contracting with clients.

As well as the differing locations of supervisor and supervisee, the location of the server for the platform used to communicate between them may be different again from the counties where either are based. This has been a source of some confusion, highlighting the new legal frontiers online communications have created. The way in which Skype processes data has been recognised as potentially problematic from a therapeutic standpoint for some time (see Quashie, 2013).

Many well-known sites for online work have servers based outside the EU, particularly the USA. Whilst successful passage of the EU wide General Data Protection Regulation and EU-US Privacy Shield in 2016 may help bring some clarity to this notoriously murky legal field, the UK's impending withdrawal from EU may create new issues which cannot at present be foreseen. As this is likely to remain a fluid topic for some time, regularly checking new ICO guidance is advised. The uncertainty around the location of their servers – and therefore what legal jurisdiction that information is in – poses another. This also highlights the importance of asserting clearly the country your practice is based in and laws to which it is subject.

Further reading on data security

ICO: UK's independent authority for information rights, providing guidance on –

o   What is data
o   Preparing for the General Data Protection Regulation (GDPR)
o   Anonymisation:managing data protection risk code of practice (https://ico.org.uk/)

PW Training: a wide selection of resources discussing and assessing data security by Pip Weitz www.pwtraining.com/resources-for-working-online/security-confidentiality-online/

Online Therapy Institute: Information on HIPAA compliant platforms available from: http://onlinetherapyinstitute.com/2011/03/01/videoconferencing-secure-encrypted-hipaa-compliant/

Resources

Part of our role as supervisors is to be able to signpost the supervisee to services and resources which support their development and support their clients. Without local knowledge, it may not be realistic, even with regular research, to aim to do this to an effective level.

Care needs to be taken when contracting to consider the supervisee's own capacity to find resources: Are they an experienced therapist with strongly embedded knowledge of local and national services? Prospective supervisor and supervisee might also consider what other contacts or support the supervisee could utilise on the ground and contract with explicit apportioning of roles accordingly.

Even if local support is acknowledged and used by the supervisee, it will still be important for the supervisor to understand what resources can be accessed – are there direct equivalents to UK services a supervisor might advise a supervisee to use in onward referrals/safety plans etc. If not, how can this be managed effectively?

Contextual knowledge

The development of contextual knowledge is a thread running through all preceding headings. The complexity of what it amounts to can feel daunting: To seek to understand a culture and society – how it evolved and what factors could be affecting the supervisee and their clients as individuals, also shaped and affected by their context.

I find my training as an anthropologist invaluable both in engaging with these questions and having an academic framework from which to undertake research. I share the surprise of Gerstein, Rountree, & Ordonez (2007) that the counselling world has not engaged more with anthropological ideas. Their research leads them to conclude that "counselling may have simply overlooked or minimised the entire discipline of anthropology" (Gerstein, Rountree, & Ordonez, 2007, p. 397). They also suggest that "the strong focus on the individual in therapy may leave counsellors" (by extension, supervisors) "resistant to an approach built on understanding social context" (Gerstein, Rountree, & Ordonez, 200,7 p. 397).

This strikes me as a potential vulnerability in online supervision, where communicating through a virtual interface, our isolation can be amplified, leading us into unhelpful or dangerous levels of fantasy (see Suler, 2004).

From within the therapeutic field, the schools of social constructionist and postmodern therapy may provide some valuable perspectives. Where Gonzalez et al speak of the therapist, making "every effort to learn the culture of the client as the client sees it" (Gonzalez, et al, 1994, p. 519) one might substitute "therapist" for "supervisor". However, they go on to acknowledge that, "Seeing truths as fluid, and thus always changing, may be a particularly knotty problem" (Gonzalez, et al, 1994, p. 522).

This sentence might strike at the heart of the tension between our roles as supervisors/therapists to sit alongside our supervisees/clients in their world and our responsibilities as professionals, trusted to identify legal and ethical boundaries – the collision of the outer and inner worlds in the therapeutic process. As Shurts (2015) describes, even in a school of therapeutic thought "based on the assumption that there is no universal 'truth' in the world [...] there are times when prescriptive approaches are vital" (Shurts, 2015, pp. 4–7).

These approaches may help us broaden our outlook, make our questions more relevant and searching perhaps, but return us once more to the stand-off implicit in the BACP guidance at the start of this chapter: Where do we stand if the ethical and legal requirements of our context collide with those of our supervisees'?

Conclusion

"There is no central database of what is allowable country by country" (Anthony, 2015, p. 39). This inevitably raises the question: "why not?" The challenges of such a venture are apparent of course. Yet, as the online field grows, it would seem both the obvious solution and one more easily achieved by a community who already understand rhizomatic, peer-led online communication.

A number of international online counselling organisations already exist, as well as a burgeoning field of academic research into the internationalisation of face-to-face psychological therapies. I would suggest that the ability of larger organisations (some listed in further resources below) to reach and mobilise a wide cross section of therapists from across international boundaries would make them the appropriate setting to continue this work.

Such a body could bring networks of people together to work on and maintain what is primarily a complex information sharing exercise. UK online therapy organisation ACTO is developing an international role on their executive and moves like this should be encouraged to promote awareness and discussion on cross border practice. Ultimately, this must present as a more sustainable and consistent long-term venture than our current isolation.

Just as online therapy is now widely recognised as a specialism, needing additional training and experience, (Anthony & Goss, 2009, p. 5) international online therapy (and supervision) should be regarded as a further level of specialist work, requiring further training and consideration of the complex additional challenges, as well as wonderful opportunities it offers.

There is an important distinction to be made between engaging with cultural nuance – to be understood, contained, and adapted – and legal and regulatory differences; which may form implacable barriers to safe and ethical work. With careful thought and research, however, many of these barriers can be safely managed. The exciting complexities of international supervision richly reward the investment of time and energy it requires of us.

Reflective questions

This chapter focusses on supervising an internationally based supervisee working with local clients. You might also consider:

o   Working with a UK based supervisee who begins offering counselling to international clients – what awareness of factors in international online therapy might you need to support and advise your supervisee appropriately?

o   A supervisor based in country A, working with a supervisee in country B, whose client is based in country C – what additional challenges, perhaps from a regulatory and legal standpoint might this present?

o   Working with a UK national, based in an international context with/without local clients. Whilst some of the immediate challenges of language might be alleviated, what other challenges might occur? Consider how the "false consensus effect" (see Leong & Ponterotto, 2003, p. 392) might be reinforced between non-indigenous actors in an alien context (something to also consider further when working internationally in an organisational context.)

Additional resources

Suggested framework for working with an internationally based supervisee

---

Consider your opportunities to research independently in the supervisee's context

o   This will involve considering the balance of:
  o   your language competency
  o   the accessibility of information (is it online or available to you by other means?)
  o   access to local (ideally therapeutically trained) contacts, whether through personal networks or professional international organisations Through research, you will need to ensure that any potential clashes between legal and ethical practices are carefully considered and any identified problems resolved or managed through clarification with relevant regulatory bodies and the supervisee before contracting.

Offer a pre-contracting information sharing interview

o   This provides an opportunity to glean contextual information on many of the points raised in this chapter and calibrate mutual understanding with the supervisee.

Allow more time for contracting

o   It may be prudent to take more time in finalising the supervision contract. For example, allowing for contract modifications to session length and format as language usage becomes clearer.
o   Signpost this expectation clearly at first contact, where the preliminary sessions may be contracted, but under review before a final contract is agreed.

Consider additional support networks available to the supervisee

o   The supervisor would need to consider the local support network available to the supervisee and consider and contract around areas of knowledge and support the supervisor may not be best placed to assist with (e.g. local resources).

Allow more time for research

o   The supervisor should expect to spend extra time researching, potentially considerably more than with a UK based supervisee. This may carry cost implications for the supervisor, which should be considered before committing to work with the supervisee.

Worksheet – questions to consider when contracting with an international supervisee

Language   Notes/other questions:

Is the supervision being carried out in a different language to the counselling work and/or not the supervisee's first language?
Consider:
o how much content can be covered in sessions
o Medium used for supervision
o Translation of transcripts
o How you can conduct research in this language

Regulations & qualifications   Notes/other questions:

o Is the supervisee qualified to their country's standards and allowed to practice?
o What equivalency do the supervisee's qualifications have to UK systems?
o Is the supervisee a member of a national therapeutic organisation?
o Is there an ethical code the supervisee abides by? Does it work in harmony with your own ethical code and regulations?
For example:
o Is the supervisee insured?
o a member of an organisational body with a complaints procedure?
o Is supervision a requirement and what requirements are made of it?
o How are counselling and psychotherapy contextualised with related professions?
o Is online therapy known and accepted? Are their limitations put on its practice?
o Does your insurance and organisational membership support working in the supervisee's country (e.g., many insurers will not cover therapeutic work in USA and Canada)

Laws   Notes/other questions:

What laws will be relevant to therapeutic practice in the supervisee's location?
e.g.,
o data law
o safeguarding and child protection
o regulation and licensing of protected professions
o How might they affect your supervision if different from UK law?
o What framework of management and enforcement do these laws operate under?
o Are there regional variations or additional laws in some territories etc.?
o What social and contextual factors may need to be understood about the enforcement of law?

Resources   Notes/other questions:

o What support is available locally for your supervisee if needed?
o What resources can she or he draw on to support or refer on a client or to seek specialist advice if needed?

Contextual knowledge   Notes/other questions:

o How will you gain an appropriate basic understanding of the social and political climate the supervisee is working in?
o What current events may be impacting on daily lives?
o What social and cultural attitudes and beliefs may contribute to unconscious assumptions about life held by:
o The supervisee
o The client(s)
o You

International therapeutic organisations

ISMHO: International Society for Mental Health Online – http://ismho.org/
EAC: European Association for Psychotherapy – www.europsyche.org/
EAP: European Association for Counselling – http://eac.eu.com/

See also –
ACTO: Association of Counsellors and Therapists Online – https://acto-org.uk/

Further Resources for Data Security and International Therapeutic Organisations

ICO: UK's independent authority for information rights, providing guidance on –

o   What is data
o   Preparing for the General Data Protection Regulation (GDPR)
o   Anonymisation: managing data protection risk code of practice (https://ico.org.uk/)

PW Training: a wide selection of resources discussing and assessing data security by Pip Weitz www.pwtraining.com/resources-for-working-online/security-confidentiality-online/

Online Therapy Institute: Information on HIPAA compliant platforms available from: http://onlinetherapyinstitute.com/2011/03/01/videoconferencing-secure-encrypted-hipaa-compliant

---

Web resources

Codice Penale (Italian Penal code) (2016). Available online at: www.brocardi.it/codice-penale/. Accessed on 22nd January 2016.

ICO (2012). What is Data: Determining what information is "data" for the purposes of the DPA. Available online at: https://ico.org.uk/media/for-organisations/documents/1609/what_is_data_for_the_purposes_of_the_dpa.pdf. Accessed on 22nd January 2016.

Montero, A., Jay, A., Owen, G., & Korintus, M. (2014). Innovative practices with marginalised families at risk of having their children taken into care. Comments paper – European Social Network (ESN) Peer Review on innovative practices with marginalised families. Venice (2014). Available online at: www.esn-eu.org/publications/index.html?&p=2. Accessed on 10th January 2016.

Quashie, R. (2013). Skype and HIPAA: The vexing question. *Tilt Magazine issue 3(3)* 2013: 41–47. Available online at: https://issuu.com/onlinetherapyinstitute/docs/tiltissue14/42. Accessed on 7th July 2016.

SAFE CIC (2015). Safeguarding whilst working overseas. Available online at: www.safe childuk.info/Charity/workingoverseas.html. Accessed on 22nd January 2016.

Saulini, A. (Ed.) (2002). The rights of children in Italy. Perspectives of the third sector. Supplementary report to the United Nations. Available online at: www.gruppocrc.net/IMG/pdf/Italy_ngowg_report_GRUPPO_CRC_EN_-2.pdf. Accessed on 12th January 2016.

UK Government Policy Paper (2014). Safeguarding children and young people. Available online at: www.gov.uk/government/publications/safeguarding-children-and-young-people/safeguarding-children-and-young-people. Accessed on 19th January 2016.

Great Britain (2015). Serious Crimes Act 2015. Available online at: www.legislation.gov.uk/ukpga/2015/9/contents/enacted. Accessed on 23rd January 2016.

References

Alberta, A. & Wood, A. (2009, May). A practical skills model for effectively engaging clients in multicultural settings. *The Counselling Psychologist, 37(4)*: 564–579.

Anthony, K. (2009). Technology and data protection. In: S. Goss & K. Anthony, (Eds.), *Technology and Counselling in Cyberspace.* London: Palgrave Macmillan.

Anthony, K. (2015). Training therapists to work effectively online and offline within digital culture. *British Journal of Guidance & Counselling, 43(1)*: 36–42.

Anthony, K., & Goss, S. (2009). *Guidelines for Online Counselling and Psychotherapy including Guidelines for Online Supervision (3rd edn).* Lutterworth: British Association for Counselling & Psychotherapy.

Anthony, K., Goss, S. & Nagel, D (2014) Developing ethical delivery of cross border services. In: P. Weitz (Ed.), *Psychotherapy 2.0.* London: Karnac.

Benbenishty, R., Davidson-Arad, B., Lopez, M., Devaney, J., Spratt, T., Koopmans, C., Knorth, E. J., Witteman, C. L. M., Del Valle, J. F., & Hayes, D. (2015). Decision making in child protection: An international comparative study on maltreatment substantiation, risk assessment and interventions recommendations and the roles of professionals' child welfare attitudes. *Child Abuse and Neglect, 49*: 63–75.

Bertotti, T., & Campanini, A. (2013). In: P. Welbourne & J. Dixon, (Eds.), *Child Protection and Child Welfare: A Global Appraisal of Cultures, Policy and Practice.* London: Jessica Kingsley.

Bessant, J. (2011). International law as remedy: When the state breaches child protection statutes. *Child & Youth Services, 32*: 254–275.

Bond, T. (2015). *Good Practice in Action 047: Ethical Framework for the Counselling Professions Supplementary Guidance: Working Online.* Lutterworth: BACP.

Chang, J. (2013). A contextual-functional meta-framework for counselling supervision. *International Journal of Advanced Counselling, 35*: 71–87.

Charura, D. (2014). Lost in translation – meeting the challenges of language and regional customs when working online, cross-border without visual cues. In: P. Weitz (Ed.), *Psychotherapy 2.0*. London: Karnac.

Collins, S. & Arthur, N. (2010). Culture-infused counselling: A model for developing multicultural competence. *Counselling Psychology Quarterly, 23(2)*: 217–233.

Costa, B. (2014). Counselling in many tongues. *Therapy Today, 25(4)*.

Crockett, S. & Hays, D. (2015, December). The Influence of supervisor multicultural competence on the supervisory working alliance, supervisee counseling self-efficacy, and supervisee satisfaction with supervision: A mediation model. *Counselor Education & Supervision, 54*.

Despenser, S. (2011). *What is Supervision?* Lutterworth: BACP

Georgiadou, L. (2015). "I was seeing more of her": international counselling trainees' perceived benefits of intercultural clinical practice. *British Journal of Guidance & Counselling, 43(5)*: 584–597.

Gerstein, L., Rountree, C., & Ordonez, A. (2007). An anthropological perspective on multicultural counselling. *Counselling Psychology Quarterly, 20(4)*: 375–400.

Gonzalez, R et al (1994) The Multicultural Perspective in Psychotherapy: A Social Constructivist Approach. *Psychotherapy, 31(3): 515–524*

Gray, J. (2015). Counsellors without borders. *Therapy Today, 26(2)*.

Great Britain (1998). The Data Protection Act. London: Stationery Office.

Goss, S. & Anthony, K. (2009) The need for and barriers to international regulation. In: S. Goss & K. Anthony (Eds.), *Technology and Counselling in Cyberspace*. Palgrave Macmillan: London.

Johansson, I. (2010). The multicultural paradox: The challenge of accommodating both power and trust in child protection. *International Social Work, 54(4)*: 535–549.

Kapasi, K., & Melluish, S. (2015). Language switching by bilingual therapists and its impact on the therapeutic alliance within psychological therapy with bilingual clients: A systematic review. *International Journal of Culture and Mental Health, 8(4)*: 458–477.

Leveille, S. & Chamberland, C. (2010). Towards a general model for child welfare and protections services: A meta-evaluation of international experiences regarding the adoption of the Framework for the Assessment of Children in Need and Their Families (FACNF). *Children and Youth Services Review, 32*: 929–944.

Leong, F. & Ponterotto, J. (2003). A Proposal for internationalizing counseling psychology in the United States: Rationale, recommendations, and challenges. *The Counseling Psychologist, 31(4)*: 381–395.

Ng, K., & Noonan, B. M. (2012). Internationalization of the counseling profession: Meaning, scope and concerns. *Int J Adv Counselling, 34*: 5–18.

Ng, K., & Smith, S. (2012). Training level, acculturation, role ambiguity and multicultural discussions in training and supervising international counseling students in the United States. *International Journal of Advanced Counselling, 34*: 72–86.

Orr, P (2010). Distance supervision, research, findings and considerations for art therapy. *The Arts in Psychotherapy*, 37: 106–111

Remley, T. P., Bacchini, E., & Krieg, P. (2010). Counseling in Italy. *Journal of Counseling & Development, Winter, 88*.

Robinson, B., Bradley, L. J., & Hendricks, C. B. (2000). Multicultural counselling supervision: A four-step model toward competency. *International Journal for the Advancement of Counselling, 22*: 131–141.

Sangganjanavanich, V. & Black, L. (2009). Clinical supervision for international counselors-in-training: implications for supervisors. *Journal of Professional Counseling: Practice, Theory, and Research, 37(2)* Fall/Winter: 52–65.

Shurts, W. M. (2015). Infusing postmodernism into counseling supervision: Challenges and recommendations. *The Journal of Counselor Preparation and Supervision, 7(3).*

Stannard, R. (2013). International registry of counsellor education programs: CACREP's contribution to the development of counseling as a global profession. *Journal of Counseling & Development, 91* January: 55–70.

Suler, J. (2004). The online disinhibition effect. *CyberPsychology & Behavior, 7(3):* 321–326.

Walsh, S. D. (2014). The bilingual therapist and transference to language: Language use in therapy and its relationship to object relational context. *Psychoanalytic Dialogues, 24(1):* 56–71.

Wright, J. & Griffiths, F. (2010). Reflective practice at a distance: using technology in counselling supervision. *Reflective Practice, 11(5):* 693–703.

Zack, J. S. (2008). How sturdy is that digital couch? Legal considerations for mental health professionals who deliver clinical services via the internet. *Journal of Technology in Human Services, 26(2–4):* 333–359.

Chapter 12

Supervision guidelines: online supervision and supervision online – what's the difference?

Philippa Weitz

Who is this chapter written for? A clarification on roles and contexts

Who might need to read this chapter? The short answer is psychological thera-pists, which amounts to around 100,000 practitioners in the UK alone. In this figure, I include anyone working as a counsellor, psychotherapist, psychologist, psychiatrist or other qualified person using counselling or psychotherapy methods for therapeutic purposes.

Are we talking about face-to-face therapists who receive their supervision online? Or are we talking about supervision of therapists who work therapeuti-cally online? Actually, the answer is both, as summarised in Figure 12.1 below.

We can see from this chart that the common denominator in all four quad-rants is the possibility of online work, often with some cross-over between them. Which quadrant(s) do you fit in? A, B, C, or D, or maybe a mixture if you have different forms of supervision?

I find it easier to grasp these groupings in a visual way. And in reality not every-one fits perfectly into each of these boxes, and some may cross-over. The outcome of this chart detailing possible supervisory groups using online supervision mean that this chapter actually is relevant to a far larger readership than might originally be expected and that any supervisor or supervisee using an online method for delivering or receiving their supervision will find this chapter useful. Jones and Stokes (2009) identify the same possible uses of supervision online (A and C in Figure 12.1), and online supervision (B and D in Figure 12.1).

With reference to supervisees, group (C), face-to-face therapists (supervisees), who may currently be the majority (no figures available for this), receive their supervision online. There is an additional sub-set in this group where this might involve a blend of supervision of face-to-face and online work.

The second group (D) of supervisees are therapists working therapeutically online. It is likely that they are already receiving their supervision online as dem-onstrated in Figure 12.1.

The consequence of these opening points is that this chapter is relevant to all those who identify in any of the four quadrants in Figure 12.1. and that *the online context is the unifying factor in all four quadrants*. This may constitute quite a large number of psychotherapists and counsellors, many of whom will not have

	Supervision online		Online supervision	
Type of supervisors	**A: *Face-to-face* supervisors** (A supervisor who supervises online the work of supervisees working face-to-face with clients)		**B: *Online* supervisors** (A supervisor who is qualified to supervise online the work of online therapists)	
	Possible methods of delivering supervision to supervisees working with *face-to-face* clients:		**Possible methods of delivering supervision to supervisees working with *online* clients:**	
	Face-to-face	*Online*		*Online*
Type of supervisees	**C: *Face-to-face* supervisees** (A therapist who works face-to-face with clients)		**D: *Online* supervisees** (A therapist who works online with clients)	
	Possible methods of receiving supervision for those therapists working with *face-to-face* clients		**Possible methods of receiving supervision for those therapists working with *online* clients**	
	Face-to-face	*Online*		*Online*

Figure 12.1 Possible methods of delivering and receiving supervision and types of supervisor

trained to work therapeutically online, and may have never seen the *BACP Online Counselling and Therapy Guidelines* (Anthony and Goss, 2009) which include a substantial and useful section on online supervision, or the more recent *BACP Supplementary Guidance for Working Online* (Bond, 2015).

Thinking about different groupings, we are generally clear what working therapeutically online is, and the consequent online supervision. I recently coined the expression *digital psychotherapy* to cover a much wider spread than just those working therapeutically online. Pollecoff and Chalfont (2014) show in their case study chapter in *Psychotherapy 2.0* (Weitz, 2014) how digital impacts both face-to-face and online consulting rooms. All counsellors and psychotherapists are impacted by some aspect of the digital world, whether it is through a face-to-face client sharing publicly via social media the content of their couple counselling, or it is the constant interruption of the client's mobile phone during sessions, or the emails between you and a client. The digitalising of psychotherapy has changed the landscape of counselling and psychotherapy forever, probably bringing the biggest change since Freud. Groups A and C in Figure 12.1 will certainly count in this digital psychotherapy definition.

Turning to ethical guidelines, the *BACP Ethical Framework* (Bond, 2016) asks us in the "Good Practice" section (paragraph 59, Supervision) to review this framework and its application to our work with clients at least once a year in supervision.

To give some texture to the chapter, I will begin Part one with a brief case study. John will pop up regularly throughout the chapter. Of course, he is a fictional- ised character and precisely because it is this that we'll all recognise elements of ourselves and our clients in this case study. Part two sets out the definitions, purposes, and role of online supervision. Part three covers an organisation's point of view, Part four the individual's point of view as either supervisor or supervisee and in Part five, I shall look at the specific guidelines for online supervision and set out what I believe to be the important elements to include in any guidelines for online supervision. The mechanics of online supervision, and its benefits and weaknesses, are covered by other chapter authors.

Part one: John, a case study

Recently, working as an online supervisor, Mary, received an email from a psy- chotherapist, John, who was looking for some online supervision. He had under- gone some training (not with Mary) to work online in which he said the following, attempting to address the robustness of his thinking about security and confiden- tiality and justifying why he didn't need any further training:

> Of course with clinical work I think of the email provider – so my clinical email account is through Fastmail in Australia because of its privacy policies. Clients of course are welcome to email from google or Microsoft products with all the dangers entailed there. I do make clear that I don't discuss clini- cal material over email just to avoid them sending long one-sided messages.

And part of Mary's reply included:

> You might want to check whether an Ozzie email account is acceptable in Europe under principle 7 of the Data Protection ACT 1998 principles and the EU's General Data Protection Regulation which the UK is signing up to despite Brexit, or whether there is a privacy shield arrangement between Australia and the EU. You should also investigate the Australian laws about data protection as they are different to EU rules. The new GDPR is similar to the ICO's data protection principles but adds a new principle, accountability and this is going to challenge all of us.
>
> Secondly, to be honest there is little point in worrying about securing your email unless you can secure your client's email. It would be like having Bank of England security, but leaving the safe door open. You can't control what your client does so I never use email for anything confidential at all, instead I give (via a separate method preferably) the client a password and then send all correspondence as a password protected file. The alternative is to use an asynchronous messaging system via a secure platform which is fully compli- ant for therapeutic work in the UK [...] but not all clients are prepared to install new software that this might require.

Reflective questions

Topics you may wish to think about regarding this email exchange:

1) In your opinion, had John read any online guidelines?
2) Was John demonstrating with "Good Practice" as described by the *BACP Ethical Framework* (Bond, 2016, pp. 5–17)?
3) Had John checked the requirements of the Data Protection Act 1998 and the General Data Protection Regulation 2016 (GDPR) and in particular principles 7 (security) and 8 (international)?
4) What issues might John wish to approach differently?
5) Do you think he has a supervisor who is qualified to work online?
6) Do you think he had undergone any training to work online therapeutically?

Part two: definitions, purposes and role of online supervision and supervision online

What guidelines for online supervision and supervision online exist?

Both Jones and Stokes (2009) and Anthony and Merz Nagel (2010) highlighted the lack of research, literature, and guidelines concerning online supervision. Not enough has changed regarding this despite seven years passing since these comments were made. This chapter addresses the issue of guidelines. Chapter two explores research into online supervision.

There are already at least two guidelines, in the UK, which refer to online supervision, both produced by the British Association for Counselling and Psychotherapy:

1. *BACP Ethical Framework* (Bond, 2016). For the purposes of online supervision, you will need to read this ethical framework together with other supporting documents within the "Good practice in action" suite. I shall quote from some of these in this chapter, but it is not easy to follow the guidelines related to working online as it requires darting between different supplementary papers. And herein, I believe, lies the first difficulty.
2. *BACP 2009 Online Counselling and Psychotherapy Guidelines* (Anthony & Goss, 2009) have everything gathered in one place, and without being dogmatic or regulatory in tone. It is written in plain English which is easy to follow and understand, and leads us to understanding how to implement these guidelines. These guidelines have the most comprehensive section on online

supervision of all the guidelines, and for this reason alone remains an important tool for onliners. Because it is now seven years old there are inevitably some items that need updating. I don't believe it contradicts the *BACP Supplementary Guidance for Working Online* (Bond, 2015) in any way, though it is not used within the current suite of online guidelines. Currently UKCP has no guidelines published although there has been a lot of work behind the scenes.

What is online supervision and what does it involve?

Until this publication, there has been frustratingly little material to draw on to create an all-encompassing definition for online supervision (and supervision online), although a number of publications mention in passing online supervision for example, Anthony & Merz Nagel (2010), Jones and Stokes (2009) Weitz (2014). *The BACP Ethical Framework* (Bond, 2016) sets the tone and pace in paragraph 20 of "Good practice, working to professional standards", stating that:

> We will fulfil the ethical principles and values set out in this Ethical Framework regardless of whether working online, face-to-face or using any other methods of communication. The technical and practical knowledge may vary according to how services are delivered but all our services will be delivered to at least fundamental professional standards or better.

Whilst it doesn't say this explicitly, I understand that implicitly supervision is included within this statement's requirements.

Within the "Good practice" section (p. 5), it sets out that members and registrants of BACP are expected to commit themselves to the *Ethical Framework*, including supervision and training. The inherent words "online" or/and "face-to-face", are implicit; it is the commitment to the Ethical Framework that is important, and then within the ethical speak of the *Ethical Framework*, it is down to us to work out how to implement this within the setting/context we find ourselves.

How might we distinguish online supervision from supervision online?

In Figure 12.1, I demonstrated the difference between online supervision and supervision online. Although there is a *BACP Supplementary Guidance: Working Online* guideline (Bond, 2015), in fact the *BACP 2016 Ethical Framework* covers supervision in great detail, especially within its Good Practice and Working to Professional Standards sections. The therapist is asked and expected to apply these principles to the individual requirements of the supervision setting, be it online, face-to-face, as stated above.

The requirements for supervision are set out in the *BACP Ethical Framework* (Bond, 2016) and in addition, as online supervisors, we are required to underlay and overlay additional aspects that relate to digital and cyberspace, such as:

- Additional security and confidentiality issues
- Adapting our chosen modality to the online context
- Digital issues
- Jurisdictional issues
- Therapeutic issues
- Relational aspects to supervision online

Had therapist John read and implemented the "Good practice" section, he might have written the email to his supervisor differently. Had his supervisor read the relevant documents she might not have been supervising him without getting some training. In the *BACP Guidelines for Online Counselling and Psychotherapy*, (Anthony & Goss, 2009) section on online supervision, the authors are very clear about the need for training to work as an online supervisor:

> Supervisors who wish to supply such a service should ensure they are experienced and trained to support their online work. Supervisors who wish to supply such a service should ensure they are experienced and trained in online therapeutic work itself and have a full understanding of the issues and ethical concerns inherent in it. Supervisors must also consider the issues surrounding client consent, confidentiality and data protection/storage when offering online supervision. (p. 10)

I wonder how many supervisors delivering their supervision online to the face-to-face supervisees are even aware of this excellent document, despite the fact it has been available to BACP members via its website for seven years. The consequences are far reaching as many supervisors are unwittingly providing online supervision in one way or another; they may be working via Skype (not advised) to deliver supervision for supervisees who are working face-to-face, or the supervisor may be seeing face-to-face supervisees who are working online, all as identified in Figure 12.1.

The relevant current document, *BACP Supplementary Guidelines for Working Online* (Bond, 2015) states in paragraph 12:

> It is considered ethically desirable to receive at least some elements of regular supervision by the same method of communication that is used with clients, in order to gain direct experience of the strengths and limitations of the chosen way of working.

Those forty-two words are the only comment on online supervision within this document. For me that is a rather an oversight, even if they might be supplemented by looking at other documents within the *Ethical Framework*. For example, Bamber (2015) in a BACP document on how to choose a supervisor, covers online work in point 6.9, but for me is far too vague regarding the actual training to work as a supervisor online or online supervisor, despite pointing the reader in a number of directions.

The BACP Guidelines for Online Counselling and Psychotherapy (Anthony & Goss, 2009) stands out with its two and a half pages of densely typed print and for the moment I would urge online supervisors and supervisors working online to continuing using these guidelines until there is a newer version specifically for online supervision and supervision delivered online. ACTO (www.acto-org. uk) are currently working on new guidelines both for online therapy and online supervision, but at the point of publication it is not known when they will be published. The resulting guidelines will be highly beneficial for both the profession and provide clarity for the general public, our clients.

On the subject of training, paragraph 12 of the *BACP Supplementary Guidelines: Working Online* (Bond, 2015) states:

> Changing the method of communication with clients introduces new challenges and opportunities that can be greatly assisted by appropriate training. Good practice requires that anyone making significant differences in their practice should give careful consideration to what will be involved and have taken adequate steps to be competent in the new ways of working before offering services to clients.

Whilst the language of these two documents is quite different, the two BACP online guidelines (2009, 2015) do seem to both recommend some training before working or supervising online.

In our case study John seems to have overlooked some important guidance, but actually his supervisor, Mary, is the one who really needs to give thought to this. When I last checked the ACTO register for supervisors qualified to work online there were only twenty-eight listed, which means that few supervisors are trained to deliver supervision online (A and C, Figure 12.1.) or online supervision (B and D, Figure 12.1). (I accept there may be some supervisors working online who are not on the ACTO register but who have developed the required competencies and skills to supervise online. Equally there may be some trained online supervisors who for one reason or another have chosen not to go on the ACTO register – but either way, the numbers are small). This includes the regular jobbing supervisor who might often or occasionally see his or her supervisees online; they all need to be aware they have liabilities and responsibilities with their supervisory role.

Fleshing these liabilities and responsibilities out, in order to avoid a situation where the therapist or supervisor finds themselves faced with a complaint about a breach of confidentiality, Steve Johnson of Oxygen Insurance advises:

> For all remote work, whether on-line or telephone, it is important that client recognises and accepts the limitations in terms of confidentiality and security

of the media before agreeing to proceed. There are also some potential issues under the Data Protection Act where servers for on-line services might be based outside the European Economic Area (EEA). The client would need to give consent if data is to be transmitted outside the EEA unless the servers are located in a "safe haven". Microsoft, the owners of Skype, for example, won't confirm their servers are a safe haven. (Johnson, 2016)

This is not about therapists and supervisors possibly finding themselves uninsured; it is more about making sure that the limitations of confidentiality are understood and accepted by all parties thereby avoiding a complaint in the event of a breach or at least being in a position to respond to any complaint with "you knew the risks and agreed to proceed anyway".

So, rule number one is always to check your working practices with your insurer – they are there to help and guide you, and would much rather do so than must deal with a complaint which is costly for everyone. Rule number two would be to check with ACTO and your professional membership body.

Part three: organisations – professional membership organisations and their role

At the time of writing, The Association for Counselling and Therapy Online (ACTO) is currently actively consulting and collaborating with the aim of putting together one set of unified online guidelines for online therapists, and, as part of that, include guidelines for online supervision. The resulting guidelines will be highly beneficial for both the profession and provide clarity for the general public, our clients.

In addition, my work in Europe has shown us just how much we're all working in a silo, and we need to start working far more closely with other European and international associations – we're in danger of reinventing the wheel. This work is critical to take into account jurisdictional issues. These are the type of knotty issues that come up in online supervision, when the supervisee has a client in say, Ecuador, Zimbabwe, India or Italy. Of course, we currently have no idea how Brexit will affect this, but it certainly won't help, for example the EU-US data privacy shield is a fine example of the EU's important role in enabling what we do. ACTO has just appointed an international director to take up this role and develop information that will be helpful around these areas.

In 2015 the United Kingdom Council for Psychotherapy (UKCP) through its education, training, and practice committee, started to think about the digital impact on psychotherapy, both within its minimum curriculum for psychotherapists and specialist online guidelines. The UKCP online guidelines, including for online supervision, are now written but not yet published.

Where does the Association for Counselling and Therapy Online (www.acto-org.uk) fit into the picture? It is "the place to go" for online therapists and online supervisors wishing to be listed within the ACTO registers, and for clients to find an online therapist. This is not an automatic listing and listing is dependent on having successfully completed training through an ACTO approved training provider.

ACTO requires all its members to be a member of a professional membership body that recognises the registrant's face-to-face qualification, such as BACP, UKCP, BCP, or BPS. It is these organisations that would deal with any complaint, not ACTO.

Together with the British Psychological Society (BPS, around 50,000 members of whom around 3,500 are in the counselling psychology division and 480 in the psychotherapy section) and the Royal College of Psychiatrists (RCPSYCH, around 3,000 members), there are around 100,000 clinicians working in psychological services in the UK (BACP 45,000 members, UKCP 7,800, ACTO ninety-two of whom twenty-eight are also listed as online supervisors), many of whom are working therapeutically online in some way.

So far, the professional membership organisations have been slow in leading the way from the front regarding working online. Many still feel it is a specialism that most face-to-face therapists do not need to engage with. I hope my earlier explanation of *digital psychotherapy* demonstrates how digital impacts on the work of every therapist (hence the reason that UKCP have included digital issues in their minimum curriculum for adult training).

Whist I appreciate the autonomy of thought and decision making provided by the *BACP 2016 Ethical Framework*, it has too many supplementary parts in my opinion. We are under such huge pressures that such detailed investigation often gets overlooked. For me, a guideline should be straightforward and complete, and easy to read, even if it might refer to other guidelines that buttress onto it. The BACP one needs too much unpacking, with each point requiring a huge amount of thinking because of the way it is written in ethical language, and I am sure I have read more of them than most! Precisely because the *BACP Ethical Framework* is couched in "Good practice", many practising counsellors and psychotherapists feel that they don't have to do anything about upgrading their knowledge of working online because it is not compulsory (I hear this all the time). Whilst this is counter-intuitive to "Our commitment to clients" in the opening sections of the *BACP 2016 Ethical Framework*, most of us are just trying to do our best and have many conflicting demands on our time, so many may take the line of least resistance. Thinking about the list of questions in the John case study, I am wondering how much training our case study John might have had.

Part four: the individual: supervisors, supervisees, and clients

Now I have another chart for you: Figure 12.2, Who's "working online"? This chart breaks the mental health profession in the UK into three groups. Group C covers all the approximately 100,000 professionals working in psychological therapies in the UK. These clinicians will be working together with patient and clients running into hundreds of thousands, maybe higher.

A very high proportion of patients and clients will have some online life (92.6 per cent or 60,273,385 UK residents are identified as internet users, individual who can access the Internet at home, via any device type and connection (*Internet Live Stats*, 2016).

The impact of these high numbers in Group C, mean that both supervisors online and online supervisors need to be fully aware and regularly updating their legal and practitioner knowledge and skills adapting to the ever changing digital and legal environment, as asked of us by the paragraphs (50–61) in the "supervision" section of the *BACP Ethical Framework* (Bond, 2016). Group C is the largest group by far, and has led me to the view that we need to address the non-therapeutic role of the internet and social media within any guidelines, "digital psychotherapy" because of the way digital matters interface with the therapeutic relationship in all contexts.

Social media is now a way of life for many of our clients, crossing boundaries and borders seamlessly. This inevitably impinges on our practice, face-to-face or online, such as how they research you before signing up for therapy, or it may be how they play out their therapy online, how they see the internet to self-medicate, how you and your clients email each other, the role and use of texting, emailing, as beautifully illustrated in Chalfont's (2014) "Penny and Liam" case study. All of these point to the need for each therapist, face-to-face or online, and their supervisor regularly to undertake training and continuing professional development in order not to fail the client.

To summarise, Group C's involvement in this aspect of guidelines regarding digital psychotherapy is paramount because they involve nearly every therapist working in the UK (let alone overseas). Even if you don't use social media yourself, you can be sure that the majority of your supervisees and their clients will. It's a fact of life for 2016 and beyond.

Turning to Group B, in Figure 12.2, in some ways, this is the most worrying group as they don't know they don't know and blindly use Skype, unsecured emails, send texts to clients, and have had no training or thought given to confidentiality and security in the digital age for psychological services. This applies to both supervisors and therapists. Whenever I run a workshop, one of my first questions is, "Are you working online at all?" Usually very few hands go up. Second question, "Do you ever send your clients emails?" Usually fifty to seventy-five per cent of hands go up. And then I leave a silence and then they all go "ah!", and that's the first stage of understanding of their digital involvement in their therapeutic work, whatever the context.

The opening scenario, John, is just one example of people in that middle band, Group B in Figure 12.2, who may have little, if any, training but are very well meaning.

What concerns me with this Group B is that their supervisors appear to have little knowledge of the various guidelines or what they mean in practice for both them and their supervisees. I have already discussed in detail above the various frameworks and guidelines that each require practitioners to consider carefully

100,000

Approximate
numbers of
mental health
professionals in
the UK based on
professional
bodies'
published
membership
numbers

A

B

C

**ONLINE THERAPY /
SUPERVISION**

1% – 3%

TRAINED & QUALIFIED TO WORK
THERAPEUTICALLY ONLINE

"I only do a little Skype"

60 – 90%

COUNSELLING / SUPERVISION
RECEIVED ONLINE + PROVIDING
THERAPY / SUPERVISION ONLINE
NO TRAINING TO WORK ONLINE

DIGITAL PSYCHOTHERAPY

Indirect involvement in both face to
face and online practices through social
media, online self-medication, APPS for
self help, google listings, chat rooms,
blogging, twitter, emailing and texting)

99%+

YOU AND YOUR CLIENT

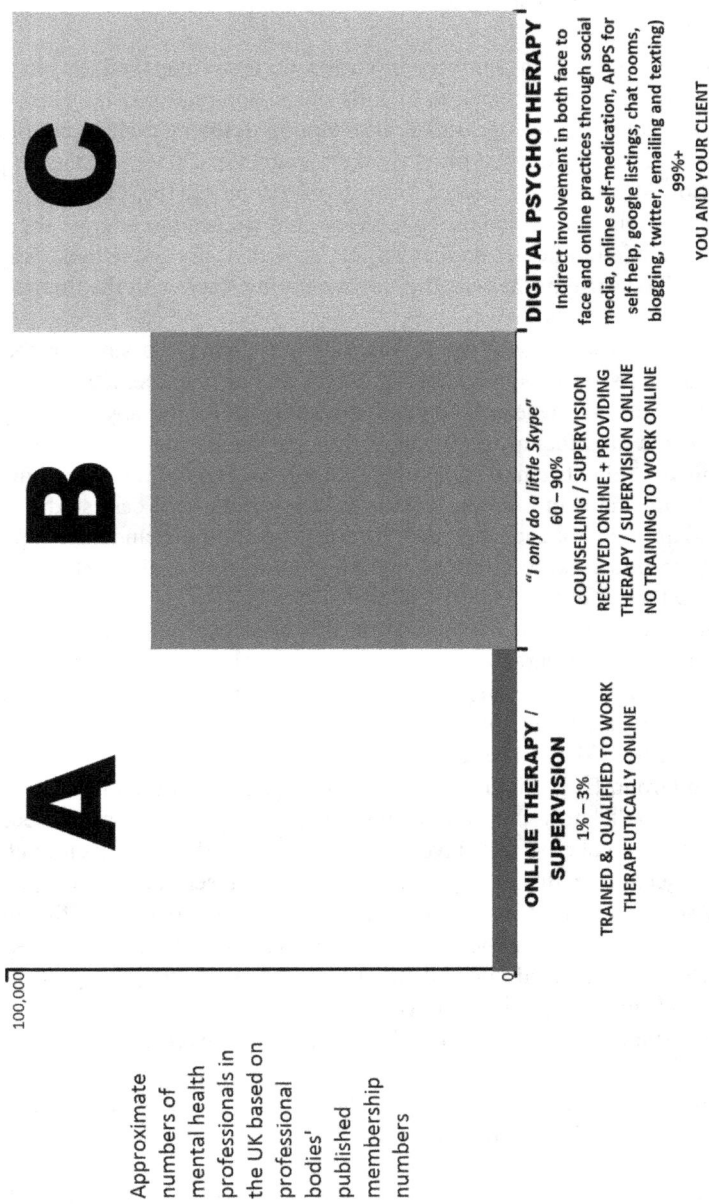

Figure 12.2 Digital psychotherapy and supervision online psychotherapy and supervision (not drawn to scale and
numbers only approximate)

how they may best receive supervision for their practice and ensure that the supervisor is experienced and trained in online work and has a full understanding of the legal and security issues, the ethical concerns and the impact for the therapeutic alliance, however this might be worded.

To summarise this section, we need to migrate to a consensus agreement amongst the online profession. Some therapists may believe working online is simply a matter of turning on their webcam, despite the widespread requests for counsellors and supervisors to undertake training before taking on these new media.

The third group, Group A in Figure 12.2, are well trained, adhere to BACP/UKCP/BPS/other professional bodies, members of ACTO and adhere to the ACTO online guidelines. They are trained to be reflective about all matters relating to working professionally therapeutically online, and are likely to have in place online supervision arrangements. But they are probably around one to three per cent of mental health professionals in the UK, and I'm probably being generous here!

As a conclusion, there is a huge mismatch between the long available online guidelines (BACP and other organisations), and the actual practice of therapists and supervisors. Equally there is a huge mismatch between the level of training and those who have no training – probably around ninety-seven per cent of therapists and supervisors have no training to work online, despite BACP guidelines encouraging every one of us to get this training and making it available through ACTO approved training providers.

BACP has recently, as part of its *Ethical Framework*, put together a whole suite of documents that are really helpful, but, in my opinion, somehow many are not engaging with these or "hearing" what they advise. As therapists, we need to provide care that is fit for 2017, where digital natives are now old enough to be training as therapists. The NHS has a major strategy to digitalise much of its care; we need to be thinking this way too. The UKCP minimum curriculum has included important requirements for every pre-qualification trainee with regard to digital matters, security, and confidentiality, which is an excellent example and really refreshing.

Part five: supervision guidelines – online supervision and supervision online fit for the future

In Figure 12.1, I distinguished between online supervision and supervision online. In Figure 12.2, I set out a breakdown of how therapists are involved digitally in psychological therapies. The outcome of both these charts is that any online supervision and supervision online guidelines need to apply to virtually everyone working therapeutically in mental health in a psychotherapeutic setting.

Any guidelines that we develop in the future need to take digital issues and formats into account, be a joint collaboration of professional membership bodies working together, and a consensus amongst online therapists and supervisors.

There will need to be a more overt presentation of these guidelines rather than finding them quietly embedded in other paperwork. We currently have a situation where only twenty-eight online supervisors are listed by ACTO as qualified to do the work required within the guidelines, whilst over ninety per cent of our clients are likely to be active digitally and more and more drawn to receive at least some of their therapy online, with the consequence that supervision will need to be delivered online. This is a terrible mismatch by any standards.

We urgently need clear online guidelines, buttressed by a career path provided by, for example but not only, ACTO, for the training of online therapists and supervision (this is currently being worked on), to send the right message both to the profession and the general public about the effectiveness of online therapy, the robustness of training for both online therapists and supervisors and a general public who know where to go when they need to seek out psychological help.

A lot changes in five years, and this means that we need guidelines for both online therapy and online supervision/supervision online that guide us and are fit for at least the next five years, taking us say to 2022.

What needs to be in guidelines for online supervision and supervision online? This is, of course, relevant equally to supervisors and supervisees. Here's a list of what could be included in any future negotiated guidelines for online supervision and supervision online:

1) Definitions

    A definition of "online supervision and supervision online".

2) Formats

    What formats might we as online supervisors use, and what a supervisee and their clients might need do and know about these formats.

3) Technological competence, digital and technology provision

    These issues include practitioners' competence with the technology, and the importance of having appropriate software, internet connectivity and knowledge.

4) Security and confidentiality

    These issues include the Information Commissioner's Office and the Data Protection Act 1998 (and its various amendments), GDPR, EU (and post Brexit) regulations, the transfer of data, having sufficient safeguards on your computer including firewalls and virus checkers, encryption, privacy, password protection, the use of technology which complies for use in the UK, choice of online platform, as well as the many aspects of confidentiality and security as they relate to therapeutic work, including the implantation of a social media policy, information pack and contract for online clients/patients.

5) The law

Any online supervision or supervisor working online will need to update regularly their legal knowledge pertaining to digital matters, including EU/UK and international law about jurisdiction, but also about safeguarding, distance selling laws, etc.

6) Responding to any breach of security or privacy

This includes setting out how to identify breaches of security or privacy and what to do if something goes wrong and how it might be remedied.

7) Working with vulnerable clients and arrangements for emergencies

Guidance for working with vulnerable clients, working out client groups that therapists might not wish to work with, and setting out arrangement for emergencies and death.

8) The rules around jurisdiction and working cross border

This covers both where the practitioner is professionally "resident" and also the client, and need to reference the Data Protection Act 1998, Schedule 1 The Data Protection Principles (ICO, 2016), which under Principle 8 considers jurisdiction issues. Both Brexit and the more recent EU-US Privacy Shield (effective from 12 July 2016) will need to be taken into account. Other issues will require checking that an insurer will cover you to work abroad (and check exceptions). Other considerations include diversity, culture and language.

9) The role of social forums for clients

As already covered in point three above, a social media policy will need to consider the role and usage of such forums, and consider how many online support services are operating, such as Big White Wall. I would expect these to grow over the next few years – we already see many examples of free or cheap online support available, and perhaps this is one of the strongest growth areas.

10) Insurance

The requirement to be insured to work online and cross borders and to be aware and understand the exclusions.

11) Training as both an online therapist and online supervisor, and supervisor online

In addition to the trainings that are suitable, currently working therapeutically and online supervision are viewed as a post-graduate training specialisms, but I can see this eroding over the next few years with the arrival of digital natives into the final stages of counselling and psychotherapy trainings.

12) Supervision

Clarity on the distinction between online supervision and supervision online, together with what constitutes a qualified online supervisor and how this might be qualitatively different from face-to-face supervision.

13) The role of social media

Clarity on the definition of social media and guidance about what social media is and is not suitable to be used by therapists, and how they may delineate their private and professional lives.

14) A list of useful resources

Guidelines can never cover every eventuality, but provide a framework. Buttressing resources would be a useful appendix to a future guideline.

15) Verification of both therapist and practitioner

Verification of both clients and therapists is a topic which divides the therapeutic online community. The decision on verification will no doubt depend on your organisation and the type of clients you are working with. How might this fit with services providing anonymous support?

16) Informed consent and contractual arrangements

Both an information pack (providing the informed consent to the client) and having a written contract are "*de rigueur*" online, whereas in face-to-face work it is less common as a written contract.

17) Delivery of supervision

It is high desirable for supervision to be delivered online for those supervisees working therapeutically online. If supervision is to be delivered online for those therapists working face-to-face they'll need to have resolved their understanding of *BACP 2015 Supplementary Guidelines Working Online*, (Bond, 2015) where it states that "it is considered ethically desirable to receive at least some elements of regular supervision by the same method of communication that is used with clients".

18) Choosing a model for supervision

Supervisors and supervisees are encouraged to think through their model for online supervision. For example, a possible model might be Inskipp and Proctor's (2001) process model, these summarising as normative (managerial aspects), formative (training and learning aspects) and restorative (emotional support aspects). To these we need to add the digital aspect to create an adapted online model for supervision.

19) Online payments

Security issues require us to think of robust payment systems and how we set about our accounting whilst maintaining confidentiality.

20) Consideration of a number of competing aspects

We need to consider in any supervisory relationship the legal, ethical, practical, digital, and clinical/relational aspects both within the relationship and within the client work that is discussed.

21) The management of boundaries online

Boundaries are far more difficult to maintain online because of the nature of social media, but also because the current online therapist community is so small, meaning that there are a number of dual roles. Having a clear register of interests such as ACTO has set up for its directors will help minimise this issue, but these are issues that will regularly need to be taken to online supervision.

22) Online platforms

A difficult topic with many sticking to Skype as the platform of choice, although this seems entirely unnecessary as it does not fully comply with the ICO's server storage regulations for the EU, and other complying platforms are easily and cheaply available (e.g., zoom.us, sylo). In all cases you should ensure that any online platform for therapeutic work online is secure and from a reputable company and complies with the "DPA data principles" (ICO, 2016) and GDPR. With the arrival of mental health platforms, such as Dr Julian where the platform manages the therapist's practical arrangements, this takes much of the responsibility away from the therapist. These new platforms will require a certain thinking about the provision and management of online supervision in this context.

Part six: discussion and conclusion

Before I started writing this chapter, I thought I was writing a chapter on guidelines for online supervision. In the writing, my ideas developed and actually, I realised that while such guidelines are very important, they account for a currently very small group. In fact, the majority of psychological therapists and their supervisors are working face-to-face but having some digital impact on their work; even if not working online, they may be receiving supervision online for face-to-face work, or have clients acting out on Facebook, as examples.

So, the chapter title got a rewrite. This is where we as a profession need to put our energies over the next five years or so as the world, our clients, our supervisees and everyone else becomes more and more digitalised. We need to encourage through training, continuing professional development, and publishing the benefits of becoming upskilled in online therapy and supervision. I hope that those working and supervising online will be inspired about the potential and growth through training to work and supervise online – I am speaking as one who has done just that, and it's the best money I ever spent!

References

Anthony, K., & Goss, S. (2009). *Guidelines for Online Counselling and Psychotherapy including Guidelines for Online Supervision (3rd edn)*. Lutterworth: British Association for Counselling & Psychotherapy.

Anthony, K. & Merz Nagel, D. (2010). *Therapy Online: A Practical Guide*. London: Sage.

Bamber, J. (2015). How to choose a supervisor. *British Association for Counselling and Psychotherapy, Good Practice in Action 008, Commonly Asked Questions Resource*. Lutterworth: British Association for Counselling & Psychotherapy.

Bond, T. (2015). *Working Online. Good Practice in Action 047: Ethical Framework for the Counselling Professions, Supplementary Guidance*. Lutterworth: British Association for Counselling Psychotherapy.

Bond, T. (2016). *Ethical Framework for the Counselling Professions*. Lutterworth: British Association for Counselling & Psychotherapy.

Chalfont, A. & Pollecoff, M. (2014). Challenges and dilemmas in the online consulting room. In: P Weitz (Ed.), *Psychotherapy 2.0: Where Psychotherapy and Technology Meet*. London: Karnac, pp. 96–97.

Davies, N. (2015). *Good Practice in Action 040 Social Media (Audio and Video) and the Counselling Professions Commonly Asked Questions Resource* Lutterworth: British Association for Counselling & Psychotherapy.

European Union. (2016). General Data Protection Regulation. Available online at: https://gdpr-info.eu/. Accessed 30 October 2017.

Great Britain (1998). The Data Protection Act. London: Stationery Office.

Information Commissioner's Office. Data Protection Act 1998, Schedule 1 The Data Protection Principles. Available online at: www.legislation.gov.uk/ukpga/1998/29/schedule/1. Accessed 8 October 2016.

Internet Live Stats. Available online at: www.internetlivestats.com/internet-users/uk/. Accessed 8 October 2016.

Johnson, S. (2016). Unpublished email correspondence between Steve Johnson and Philippa Weitz.

Jones, G. & Stokes, A. (2009). *Online Counselling: A Handbook for Practitioners*. Basingstoke: Palgrave MacMillan.

Inskipp, F., & Proctor, B. (2001). *Making the Most of Supervision, Part 1*. Twickenham: Cascade.

Weitz, P. (Ed.) (2014). *Psychotherapy 2.0: Where Psychotherapy and Technology Meet*. London: Karnac.

Wigmore, I. Social media. Available online at: http://whatis.techtarget.com/definition/social-media. Accessed 8 October 2016.

Part III

Specific contexts in online supervision

Chapter 13

Online supervision and disability

Babs McDonald

Someone recently said to me, "Online supervision and disability? That's a bit of a specialist subject!" It certainly is.

According to Department for Work and Pensions' estimates, (DWP, 2014), there are approximately 11.6 million disabled people in Great Britain. However, despite the prevalence of disability, there is very little specific information about supervision and disability, and even less when we consider it in the online context. So, it is good to be given the opportunity to explore it here.

The specific areas I thought we might consider are firstly, the subject of disability itself, then disability in the context of supervision generally, and finally, how working with disabilities might affect supervisors who work online.

In researching for this chapter, I have learnt a lot about how it feels to be a disabled person. At first this might sound strange because actually I have a disability myself. I have been hard of hearing since I was two years of age and my hearing has steadily deteriorated, especially in the last few years. However, until very recently I did not consider myself to be a disabled person and interestingly I have discovered that this is exactly how many others feel too.

For those interested in finding out more about disability, Future Learn run some excellent free six-week online courses. Two courses they run relating to disability are: "disability and a good life: working with disability" and "disability and a good life: thinking through disability".

Disability Matters is another free e-learning resource and they have a number of different online modules to assist in the understanding of disability.

Louise Smith, a lecturer at UNSW, Australia and lead educator at Future Learn says that:

> Disability results from negative interactions between someone's impairment and their societal environment. Disabling effects of society might include physical inaccessibility of spaces, exclusion from paid work, barriers to learning and education, disabling attitudes and stereotypes, etc. (Week One)

So, it is not the disability itself but other people's attitudes that define the way that a person feels about their disability. It is the prejudice, and occasionally irritation, that disabled people sometimes experience from able-bodied people. I have certainly experienced this myself and it is at these times that I feel that I have a disability.

It might be helpful to examine what is considered to constitute a disability. Often in this chapter, I will be talking from the perspective of my personal experience as a hard of hearing person. Being hard of hearing or deaf is normally classed as a disability. Other groups could include those who are blind or partially sighted; as well as any other physical or mental condition that limits a person's movements, senses, or activities. A long-term illness is also sometimes considered to be a disability and is discussed in chapter fourteen.

In a video I saw recently when completing one of the above courses, a lady explained how she had gone to two speed dating events. One was on the ground floor and she was able to access it in her wheelchair. The other was on the second floor of a building and she had to be carried up the stairs and put on a chair, leaving her wheelchair behind downstairs. You might at first, feel indignant about this; however, at this event many men came over to talk to her. Whereas when she was in her wheelchair, she said she was largely ignored. In other words, her disability was viewed as defining her and she actually had a more enjoyable time at the place which was not disability friendly. For this lady, it proved to be an enlightening, if somewhat disappointing, experience in noting how differently she was treated when viewed as an able-bodied person.

Her experience gives us some insight into why some disabled people might choose online work instead of face-to-face therapy or supervision. It means that their disability is invisible until, or unless, they wish to disclose it, perhaps when the relationship has developed and they feel safe.

In general, and in all walks of life, disabled people are often at risk of stigmatisation, of bullying and of social isolation, which may result in anxiety or depression. In addition, their disabling conditions could exacerbate their anxiety. People with a range of disabling conditions are vulnerable to being worried and anxious and, as mentioned further on in this chapter, they might not feel able to tell you this.

So, it is understandable that people with disabilities prefer not to be defined by their disability, but would like to be considered foremost as a person. The quote below from a disabled supervisee, highlights the feelings behind this quite clearly.

Were you to bring up the subject of my disability during supervision without my prompting, I would at the very least be surprised. On a deeper level, I think several things would happen. Initially I would feel offended but go with you on it out of politeness, all the while turning things over in my head which had little or nothing to do with my client. I would "humour" you. Afterwards, my reflections would once again have little to do with my clients and during the weeks between supervision sessions I would gradually become very angry and we would have to deal with this. The vital missing ingredients would be my clients. I will talk about my disability with you when it gets in the way, either on a practical level or when it is an issue within my client work. As you know, both these situations are rare. Otherwise, I simply accept that you see me as a whole person and don't treat me any differently to any of your other supervisees. Were this not the case I would feel that my clients were being overlooked in favour of my disability and that I was being discriminated against. (Page & Wosket, 2001, p. 208)

This leads us nicely on to our consideration of disability in the supervisory context generally. I would like to start with the following words, written in 1999.

Counsellors working with persons with a disability need to be encouraged to look at their attitudes, prejudices and thoughts, as do we as supervisors. It is the responsibility of the supervisor to encourage supervisees to explore these issues within the supervision context and within their own personal therapy as appropriate. This also applies to supervisors themselves. (Carroll & Holloway, 1999, p. 40)

These words were written over seventeen years ago; quite a long time in our fast-moving times and thus we might well ask ourselves if they are still relevant today. In what we like to think of as today's more enlightened world, do we still need to be reminded to look at our attitudes and prejudices? Yes, unfortunately, I think we do, since many people still define a disabled person by his or her disabilities.

Before discussing online supervision within the context of disabilities, it might be useful to understand some of the challenges that a disabled online supervisee or supervisor has faced in becoming a counsellor or supervisor in the first place.

There are many difficulties that come up in everyday life for a disabled person in an able-bodied world. With my particular disability, I struggled through my face-to-face counselling training, as sometimes my needs were not given any special consideration. At first, I was loathe to speak out about my needs, but gradually I began to realise that if I did not speak out, I would be at a great disadvantage to my learning peers.

The Fed Centre for Independent Living in Brighton and Hove conducted some interesting research about barriers and opportunities for disabled people in the area. Most of the research was about accessibility to support in their home environment, work and travel. From a therapeutic point of view, I noted that the people who took part in the research struggled with confidence and the communication of their wants and needs. The conclusion noted that, "People also felt a strong need to be valued [...] had very little choice and control in their lives [...]" (Hastie, 2012, p. 22). For me the main point that came out when reading the research was the lack of confidence to communicate what they needed. So, if a supervisee brings either their disability or their client's disability to supervision, it could be that some work around how the client/supervisee might build their confidence would be useful.

Going back to my training, I eventually found the confidence to ask for additional support. I quickly discovered that some tutors went out of their way to facilitate my learning by asking how they could help to improve the learning environment for me. Sometimes they could do nothing about the situation. An example here could be the showing of videos/DVDs without subtitles – the hard of hearing really struggle with televised speech, especially when there are background noises, such as music. One of my tutors would very kindly lend me the DVDs to listen to at home, as the sound was much clearer when I wore earphones.

Other tutors were not quite as accommodating. The learning environment for those with special needs can be fraught with difficulties that require additional work to accommodate, and sadly sometimes it is not accommodated. This is despite the amount of "banging on" about the importance of acceptance of difference and diversity, which forms part of most counselling courses these days. However, having said that, I think that within training generally, awareness is improving. The important points to bear in mind are that your disabled trainee/supervisee might not always ask for the help they need, and they may need approaching to ask whether there is anything that can be done to assist them get the most out of their sessions.

Going back to supervision, a word of caution relating to the supervisory relationship should be mentioned here though. It might be important to think about the words of Page and Wosket: "A further pitfall exists where supervisor and supervisee may become distracted from the ongoing tasks of supervision through an unwarranted emphasis on aspects of difference and diversity" (Page & Wosket, 2001, p. 211). We need to get a balance and not allow either party to be distracted from the work of supervision. Over-emphasis can result in the supervisee or client feeling "defined by their disabilities" rather than viewed as a person and I think the earlier example of the disabled supervisee illustrated this clearly.

As a hard of hearing person, I am aware that many times in my adult life, I have felt anxious in certain social situations, such as when attending conferences; in meetings or as previously written, in training. To explain, perhaps we need to think about how people with hearing loss cope with communication. Many use a combination of lip reading, hearing aids and asking people to repeat themselves. Others just suffer in silence, because they do not wish to draw attention to their disability. So, they do not ask for any concessions to be made, which can result in them feeling isolated and sometimes a little stupid. Often what those who are hard of hearing find is that people tend to come to the conclusion that they must have learning difficulties or, to put it bluntly, be a bit stupid.

Thus, my anxiety in the past has stemmed from a fear of making a fool of myself through not hearing correctly. As mentioned above, I have discovered over the years that people naturally tend to think that the hard of hearing person does not understand what is being said, when in fact it is simply a case that they cannot *hear* what is being said. The result has been that at times I have been left feeling that the person I am talking to believes that I am not very intelligent. I have had people who have, whilst looking exasperated, repeated whatever they have just said in a very over-simplified form as if talking to a very young child, even though I have explained that I am hard of hearing. It does little for one's self-esteem when people do this.

It was from this perspective, that I was immediately drawn to online counselling from the minute I began my early training. I thought that using text without having to use sound would be wonderful. Freeing, in fact, and I would feel as though I were on a level playing field

Many agencies, particularly for young people, use instant chat with their clients online, so there are plenty of opportunities to work in text alone online. In private practice, clients or supervisees who may have restricted access to face-to-face support because of physical mobility may also choose to access online services using text.

With this in mind, after I had qualified as a counsellor I immediately sought out Online Training for Counsellors Ltd (OLT), and over the next couple of years I worked my way through the general certificate in online counselling, then the diploma and eventually also the diploma in online therapeutic supervision. Thankfully most of their classes are held using instant text chat, which was perfect for my needs.

It might be helpful here to identify the possible different scenarios that may occur when considering online supervision and disability.

In *Supervision in Context* Carroll & Holloway (1999, p. 42) suggested that the "matrix of possible triads" in relation to different races/cultures developed by Lago and Thompson (1996) could be adapted when thinking about the supervisory relationship. We can develop it even further by considering it in the online context. As we are considering online supervision here, the supervisor is likely to be online but either the counsellor or client perhaps not necessarily.

Therefore, the triangle could take many different forms. For example, an able-bodied counsellor could be working face-to-face with a disabled client, supervised by an able-bodied online supervisor; or a disabled online counsellor could be consulting an able- bodied online supervisor about an able-bodied client, or

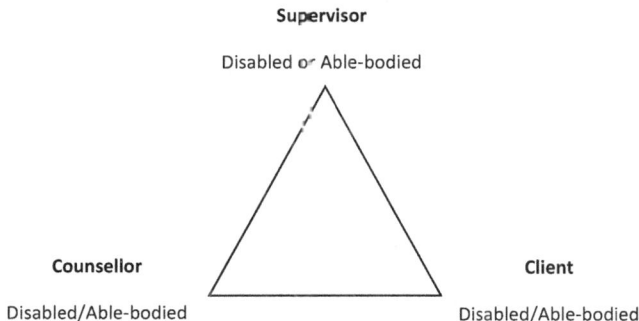

Supervisor

Disabled or Able-bodied

Counsellor   **Client**

Disabled/Able-bodied   Disabled/Able-bodied

Figure 13.1 Matrix of possible triads

any other combination of the above. Any of these scenarios might be something that needs to be given consideration in online supervision, both in terms of the issues that may arise as well as the practicalities.

In the online context, do we still need to think about the suitability of our environment? By this I mean, if we were supervising face-to-face and we had a counsellor who needed wheelchair access, we would need to give this some consideration, particularly if we worked from an upstairs room. Although we may not need to worry about this when working online, there may be other needs within the online environment. The hard of hearing for example, might find using a webcam extremely difficult, as sound does not always carry well through technology.

On the other hand, someone who is deaf might be able to access online supervision or counselling by using a British Sign Language (BSL) signing counsellor/supervisor or by using a BSL interpreter sitting in on the Skype (or other platform) session.

> This interpreter should whenever possible, be someone entirely neutral and, of course, someone who understands and pledges total confidentiality. This interpreter will be included in the counselling [or supervision] contract. (Brearley & Birchley, 1994, p. 72)

If our supervisee needs to use specialist software and equipment, we may possibly need to allow more time for a session. However, speech recognition software has greatly improved over the years and "Dragon" produced by Nuance allows hands-free interaction with ninety-nine per cent recognition accuracy the makers say, as well as being three times faster than typing, thus giving much greater freedom to people who find typing difficult. There are lots of other platforms being developed and there is also the possibility that we ourselves might need to understand how some specialist software or platform works for our supervisee or his or her client, in order to assist them to get the most out of their online supervision or counselling.

There are other possibilities in exploring different ways of working online with a disabled person. "[…] virtual reality communities [such as Second Life] can […] provide empowering experiences for some people who feel disadvantaged in real life (e.g. through physical disability, communication problems, etc.)" (Jones & Stokes, 2009, p. 91).

If you are asked to work with a disabled supervisee, or if your able-bodied supervisee is asked to work with a disabled client online, you might find yourself needing to think through some of the following questions. For example, is there a need when contracting with our supervisees or clients to know whether there are any disabilities present? Do we need to include interpreters in the contract? Why might someone choose not to disclose their disability? Could there be a reason that they have not disclosed? For example, as mentioned above, the freedom of not being defined by their disability.

When I am working online using text, I feel freed. By this I mean that unlike when I am in a face-to-face setting, I do not feel at a disadvantage to most of the people around me. Unless I choose to tell people, no-one will notice my disability because it is unseen in this context.

So other people with different disabilities could be feeling freed in just the same way. Especially if the issues they wish to talk about are not related to their disability; they can feel free to talk about anything they want without fear that they are being judged or viewed through their disability, whatever form that might take. It could be that this is the first time they have had the opportunity to not be defined by their disability. If they wish to disclose, it is their choice.

Lago and Thompson (1996) gave some suggested questions to counsellors in helping them to think about working with people from a different culture. These same questions could be relevant for us and our supervisees who are working with clients who have disabilities, when they themselves are not disabled. In other words, these could be questions to think about when working with difference and diversity generally, and in this case, disability.

Suggested questions:

1. Does the client have a right to check out the therapist before making a commitment?
2. How confident is the therapist in being open to questions from the client?
3. In such circumstances, how do you feel you would respond?
4. How much information does the therapist need to give to the client to help contribute towards a trusting relationship?
5. How is trust established between client and therapist?
6. Can you identify the range of issues [here] beyond that of establishing trust?
7. If you felt threatened or inadequate by the client/by the client's questions what would you do?

   a) refer the client elsewhere?
   b) take it to supervision?
   c) gain extra training?
   d) what else?

(Lago & Thompson, 1996, p. 105)

In concluding this chapter, I think the main points I would like to reiterate are the words from Louise Smith of FutureLearn: "Disability results from negative interactions between someone's impairment and their societal environment [...]." Like everyone else, disabled people want to be allowed the freedom to talk about whatever issues they choose to. In other words, they do not want to be defined by their disabilities.

With respect to their own disability perhaps we need to allow our supervisees to be "in charge" of when they need bring it to supervision. In respect of their clients, the same principle needs to be applied – non-directive client-centred counselling. I always like to remind myself that the only expert on myself is me and this is true for everyone. We can learn and be guided by the disabled person to bring what they want to bring and to ask for help where they feel they need it.

I think in my research, the words "defined by their disabilities" really struck a chord and felt very relevant to working online. It could be that online is the one place where a client, supervisee or supervisor can be themselves, be disability free if they so choose. For many, they have the option to disclose whenever it suits them or not at all.

In our initial contracting with supervisees, or in their contracting with their clients, we could ask whether they have any special needs. It is then up to the supervisee or client whether they want to disclose that they have a disability. If they do have special needs that they want us to accommodate then we need to check whether we can indeed facilitate these and if not, refer or signpost them on to someone who can.

The internet can be a great leveller. However, as some research conducted by Ofcom in 2013 shows, the older generation still need some education on the benefits and ease of using the internet.

> The research shows that among the youngest age group (15–34), levels of internet access are broadly comparable, regardless of whether people have a disability or not (90% compared with 93%). This increases to 94% for disabled people and 97% for non-disabled people among the more affluent in this age group.
>
> However, for older (65+) less affluent disabled people, internet access levels are at their lowest (23%) which is significantly lower than among non-disabled people of the same age and socio-economic group (37%).
>
> Across all age groups, internet ownership is 55% for disabled consumers, compared with 83% for non-disabled consumers. This can partly be explained by their older profile as half of disabled people are aged 65+. ("Younger disabled people enjoying the benefits of being online – Ofcom", 2013)

Let us hope that the use of the internet for supervision and counselling continues to grow and alongside it the specialist training that this work requires, as more and more people see the potential for working in this field.

Useful organisations

Organisations for the blind:

https://actionforblindpeople.org.uk
http://blindnewworld.org (American)

www.hertsblind.com/
www.rnib.org.uk
www.royalblind.org
www.scope.org.uk/support/families/diagnosis/visual
www.visionary.org.uk/

Organisations for the hard of hearing:

www.actiononhearingloss.org.uk/
www.bda.org.uk/
www.british-sign.co.uk/
www.hearfirst.org.uk/
www.ndcs.org.uk (For young people under 18)
www.royaldeaf.org.uk/

Organisations for disabled people:

www.learningdisabilities.org.uk/help-information/key-organisations/
www.scope.org.uk
www.ukdpc.net (United Kingdom's Disabled People's Council)
www.vodg.org.uk

Other useful resources:

Disability Matters: www.disabilitymatters.org.uk/
Dragon, voice recognition software: www.nuance.co.uk/dragon/
Online Training for Counsellors: www.onlinetrainingforcounsellors.com/

References

Brearley, G. & Birchley, P. (1994). *Counselling in Disability and Illness.* London: Times Mirror International.

Carroll, M. & Holloway, E. (1999). *Counselling Supervision in Context.* London: Sage Publications Limited.

Department for Work and Pensions (2014). Disability prevalence estimates 2011/12. Available online at: www.gov.uk/government/uploads/system/uploads/attachment_data/file/321594/disability-prevalence.pdf.

Disability and a good life: Thinking through disability – free online course. (2016). Future Learn. Available online at: www.futurelearn.com/courses/thinking-through-disability.

Disability and a good life: working with disability – free online course. (2016). Future Learn. Available online at: www.futurelearn.com/courses/working-with-disability.

Hastie, J. (2012). *Countability: Barriers and Opportunities for Disabled People in Brighton & Hove.* Brighton & Hove: The Fed Centre for Independent Living. Available online at: www.thefedonline.org.uk/countability-research-project.

Jones, G. & Stokes. A. (2009). *Online Counselling: A Handbook for Practitioners.* Basingstoke: Palgrave Macmillan.

Lago, C. & Thompson. J. (1996). *Race, Culture and Counselling*. Buckingham: Open University Press.

Page, S. & Wosket, V. (2001). *Supervising the Counsellor – A Cyclical Model*. Hove: Routledge.

Younger disabled people enjoying the benefits of being online – Ofcom. (2013). Ofcom.org.uk. Available online at: www.ofcom.org.uk/about-ofcom/latest/media/media-releases/2013/younger-disabled-people-enjoying-the-benefits-of-being-online.

Chapter 14

Using creativity in online supervision and chronic illness

Olivia Djouadi

Introduction

Chronic illnesses are a group of health-related conditions that affect millions of people worldwide therefore the possibility of having an online client with such a condition is probable. It is not only online counsellors that are reassessing how to work with these people but also online supervisors who guide counsellors through their work. According to the World Health Organisation (WHO) in 2005, thirty-five million people world-wide died from a chronic health condition and half of those were under the age of seventy (WHO. 2014). There are many millions more with chronic conditions in countries that have access to the internet so they may reach out to online groups or online counselling. Some conditions are unseen so it can be hard to describe what is going on internally. Most conditions are treated within a medical framework where emotional support can be limited or non-existent.

In this chapter, I will be reviewing the personal, social, and cultural influences that a chronic illness can have on a person and how this can affect a supervisory relationship. The supervisory framework I will be referencing is a creative model as this can assist in a diverse range of ways to help not only the supervisory relationship but also with the clients their supervisees have in their practice. It is important to note that creative supervision can be used in many modalities, as shown in *Creative Supervision Across Modalities* (Chesner & Zografou, 2014). I will also be reviewing both the concerns and advantages one can gain from the work done with those who have a chronic condition that may be affecting their emotional stability. Ben-Shahar in his book *Touching the Relational Edge* spoke of the "lifespan development process" when talking about part of the character structure (Ben-Shahar, 2014, p. 113) which can change with chronic illness. After reading this chapter, I hope you will have gained a better understanding and confidence when working as a supervisor to supervisees with chronic conditions and/or the disabled clients they care for in practice.

What is a chronic illness?

A chronic illness can be developed at any time in life, from birth like cystic fibrosis or later in life for example, cancer or dementia. There are some illnesses, like

HIV, that can be present from birth (from the mother) or occur later in life. Since there are so many illnesses, as counsellors and supervisors we will not have the same knowledge as the medical team that is working with a client with a chronic illness. Even those with the same condition cannot know what the other is experiencing without asking them. However, it is important that the illness is acknowledged from the start so it is a good idea to include on an assessment form not only questions about possible mental health conditions, but also medical conditions. Upon meeting a client either face-to-face or online, ask what needs to be done if they have a medical emergency during a session. It could be that the situation never occurs; however, it is best practice to have these details. As a result, those supervising these counsellors (and other clinicians) should discuss with their supervisees their duty of care for working with those with a chronic illness.

There are too many illnesses to list all of them in this chapter. Some of the more known conditions are mental health ones like bipolar or schizophrenia; others are medical ones such as cancer, asthma, diabetes, arthritis, epilepsy, haemophilia, multiple sclerosis, a multitude of pain disorders, Crohn's disease, COPD. Every single person needs to be acknowledged as an individual, so it is important that clients are not seen as a condition. Medications can have various effects, and people's mental stability, family dynamics, and views from the public or government can all have an effect on how well a person can function. Those who do ask for counselling may have to wait months, or even years, to be seen and for some a local counselling room is not accessible, so online counselling is a lifeline for these people.

The context of chronic illness

On an interpersonal level, there can be the views from the supervisor, the supervisee and their client which can enhance or affect the supervisory relationship. Some may be unfamiliar with chronic illness because they have not worked with them or don't know anyone with a chronic illness. Some may have their own chronic illness which they live with, as well as working in the counselling profession. Some may be afraid of illness because it is a type of unknown; illness may have its symptoms and treatments but that doesn't explain the emotional effect it may have on a person. The date of diagnosis can also impinge on the person with the illness as they may have split their life into "when I was healthy and after I got sick". Some who are born with the condition or get it during the preschool years may not be used to it, so asking is a better solution than guessing.

Some may view the chronic illness as part of them and others may feel it is something attached to them. Chronic illness is full-time; that can be a heavy burden on someone and those who care for them. Anxiety and depression are common in those with health issues, so as a supervisor it may be a good discussion to have with the supervisee. Macmillan Cancer Support outlines a range of feelings such as anxiety, depression, and loneliness (MacMillan, 2014). Jones, Fitzpatrick, and Rogers (2012) mention grief, denial, shock, anger, anguish, and depression for patients who are physically ill. These feelings are also mentioned for those with diabetes on their webpage (see www.diabetes.org.uk/Guide-to-diabetes/ Living_with_diabetes/Diabetes-burnout/).

While working with a client who has anxiety or depression, the supervisee may feel they are carrying that for the client in session. Although chronic illnesses do not pass from clients to supervisees, this emotional weight may appear for those working with them. As counsellors, it is our job to help to review those emotions so the client is more able to hold what is theirs at a later point. Anxiety can occur for the client, supervisee, and supervisor when caught in the minefield of "what ifs...". There may be psychoeducation that needs to be taught in a supervisory session which will then assist the clients to distinguish between what is medical and what is emotional. The two are interlinked and it has been found that when people are more content then medical conditions improve a little; however, I must stress counselling helps but does not cure chronic illness.

The meaning of chronic illness can be interesting as we all have our own individual thoughts. There is a big difference between, "I live with a chronic illness" and "My chronic illness might kill me" – from two people with the same illness. For some the chronic illness may be a life limiting one; however, it is important to note that clients still need to discuss the concerns that may have nothing to do with their illness. It can be that after the first session the chronic illness is barely mentioned at all; one needs to be wary of not becoming overly interested in how ill a person may be because it can make the person feel they *are* their condition. It might also be the only topic talked about because balancing life and illness is not always easy. At times two people in the client, supervisee, and supervisor relationship may have the same condition as illnesses such as cancer and diabetes. I've put the possible situations in a table to show the complexities that can occur in the relationship depending on what each person may have as a chronic illness.

As a result of many conditions being unseen, it may not be apparent who has what until a later time. The supervisor, the supervisee or the client may be a carer to someone with a chronic illness and so the worry about the person they're not presently caring for (because they're in the session) may be manifested in the room. For some people who have past trauma history or PTSD, this worry can be exacerbated so it is important to note the histories as well as present medical circumstances. Pain disorders such as fibromyalgia seem to be common for those

Table 14.1 Possible chronic illness combinations in the relationships

Supervisor	Supervisee	Client/s
Chronic illness		
	Chronic illness	
		Chronic illness
	Chronic illness	Chronic illness
Chronic illness	Chronic illness	
Chronic illness	Chronic illness	Chronic illness

with past severe trauma or traumatic stress (Scaer, 2007); however, one needs to be careful not to view a condition as proof of past trauma. These assumptions can be reviewed within the supervisory session online and if it seems an increase to monthly supervision sessions is needed, then that can be discussed between the supervisee and supervisor; this can mean meeting twice a month rather than once a month or even weekly depending on the number of clients a supervisee may have and the work involved.

Cultural aspects also play a part in the relationship as illness can be viewed in various ways depending on the family or location. Some may view illness as a part of life; some may take on huge challenges despite having a chronic illness, whereas others may consider that an illness should be cared for and the person with it should not do much. In some families, unfortunately, the person with a chronic illness may be scapegoated which can be heavy to carry. This can be difficult to resolve especially if the person with the chronic illness needs the family for support. However, we have the capacity to get additional support online if those at home cannot assist; it maybe that they need extra support as well. As online practitioners, we may know of online support agencies such as the Samaritans at www.samaritans.org/ or University Hospital Birmingham who have a list of various support groups at, www.uhb.nhs.uk/support-groups.htm, so clients can start to see a way out of where they are at present. In a supervisory relationship, the possibility of additional support can be discussed to help the clients.

Supervision model

When I work with supervisees, the creative supervision model seems to help the variety of dynamics arising when working with clients who have a chronic illness. There are a number of art forms that can be used in a supervisory session to gain better understanding of what is happening with a particular client. I find it can also help alleviate some of the concerns a supervisee may have over working with someone who has a chronic condition. The concerns can come from the discussions about health they have with their client or their own preconceived views on a given illness. In this work reflections can then be made that will assist the ongoing work or process in a given relationship. Aspects of the creative process can really help the working alliance and these connections also assist the rapport within the relationship of the supervisee and supervisor.

One way of bringing a balanced overview of the process is by using Hawkins and Shohet's seven-eyed model (Chesner & Zagrafou, 2014). This model is discussed in more detail in chapter three. These "eyes" can be accessed by using creative methods. The seven eyes are:

1. The client and how they present
2. Strategies/interventions used by the supervisee
3. Client/supervisee relationship
4. The supervisee

5. The supervisory relationship
6. The supervisor's own process
7. The wider context of the supervisee, supervisor and organisation

John Launer, as noted in the book *Inspiring Creative Supervision,* spoke of the seven Cs which can be useful to a supervisor while with their supervisee/s in Schuck & Wood (2011, p. 112).

1. Conversation
2. Curiosity
3. Context
4. Complexity
5. Caution or challenge
6. Care
7. Co-creation

Joseph Zinker (1977, p. 48) noted that clinicians who are creative have abilities that can be seen as contradictory. They can both be interested in "complexity and obscure details [...] also attracted to and seeks order". The ability to hold both these contradictions in a supervisory relationship helps to show the internal process of the supervisee and the wider picture. This is seen in other models; however, with a creative model, alternative views may also emerge that can assist the triangle of care between the supervisor, supervisee, and their clients. Creativity is found in many forms of therapy.

Much learned through discussion can be enhanced with visual stimulants and exercises that can tap into the unconscious. What is discovered can help the supervisory relationship and also assist within the relationship the supervisee may have with their own counsellor. Due to part of the unconscious being awoken, it is easy for the supervision to become therapeutic; at times a supervisor can enquire whether the supervisee might look into seeking their own counselling. As supervisors are counsellors or psychotherapists first, it can be important not to take on both roles as focus needs to be kept on the development of the supervisee and the client work. There may be times when the actual client work is limited in discussion if certain of the supervisee's feelings are on the surface. Through creativity the focus may be on feelings of sadness, frustration or excitement over achievements made both within the client work and outside. Gaining perspective over a certain feeling can help to enhance the relationship the supervisee has with their client.

Goal setting can also be enhanced by a variety of creative activities within supervision. Goal setting occurs in many areas outside of the counselling relationship with works like *The Artist's Way* by Julia Cameron (1995), where a multitude of creative possibilities help in accomplishments and tasks people have in life. I recommend clinicians read her book as well as *Creative Process in Gestalt Therapy* by Joseph Zinker, *The Therapeutic Potential of Creative Writing* by Gillie

Bolton, and *Creative Supervision Across Modalities* edited by Anna Chesner and Lia Zografou. Each creative discipline will feel right for different supervisors, and it's trial and error to find out which ones most suit the individual supervisor. One book which outlines many of these possibilities is *Inspiring Creative Supervision* by Caroline Schuck and Jane Wood with chapters reviewing various methods. I will discuss in this chapter some of the exercises that can be used to assist a supervisory relationship.

Some exercises I have found useful

1. Writing

One method I use which doesn't take too much time out of the supervision session is by noting a feeling a supervisee may be struggling with and ask them to get out a notepad and write for five minutes without stopping and not worrying about grammar or content. By doing this exercise the key to any given feeling the supervisee may be struggling with during the session may emerge. After completing the task, I will ask them to read it out because hearing what they have written can also help them to reflect on what they are going through. Bolton mentioned in her book *The Therapeutic Potential of Creative Writing* that reflective writing helps to move "onwards and upwards" from stagnation (Bolton, 1999, p. 123).

A second method I have used is similar to free association, discussed by Sigmund Freud in his lectures where he said this was a "fundamental technical rule of analysis" (Freud, 1933). I ask a supervisee to get out a piece of paper while focusing on a given tension concerning the client. Then I asked them to write any words or comments that come to mind for two minutes and I'll let them know when time is up. After this piece of work, they may have noticed a familiar theme in what has been written which can be discussed in session if they choose to do so.

2. Colours

The use of colours is quite a personal exercise as each person may have their own view on what a colour means to them. For example, red may bring a feeling of anger or passion or images of heart surgery; supervisee's may also connect certain clients to a specific colour which can be discussed in session.

Colours can also be used when discussing family dynamics of a given client. This can either be drawn on paper then photographed and sent via email or messenger, or drawn digitally. If this method is used over a number of months, the colours representing each family member may change along with the client themselves.

3. Art pieces on postcards, magazine clippings

This can be used as supervision home work. Ask a supervisee to look for a piece of art perhaps or postcards or pictures from magazines that they feel represents their client or client situation. Another method is to give the supervisee three minutes to search the Internet for art that they connect to their client. The reason I give short time periods is that for many people searching the net it can take a life of its own and may leave little time for the supervision session. Email supervision guidelines can be given; however, the supervisee is free to look for art pieces for as long as they want as it's their time. Video sessions in Skype, VSee, Zoom or others will need to have time-limited searches.

4. StoryWorld cards

This series of cards was first introduced as a creative writing tool for younger people to inspire them in numerous ways. Now they are being used in counselling and supervision to assist with the session. Each card has a theme and lots of other drawings contained within that card, which would give a supervisee a variety of items they may connect to a client situation. These can also be used in therapy so if a supervisee has really connected to these cards, they are able to buy them online (see www.templar.co.uk/brands/StoryWorld.html).

5. Psycards

These are a set of forty cards designed by Maggie Keen who was familiar with the works of Carl Jung, so designed and named the cards after the archetypes. As a result, they can be used in family discussions or to bring to the surface a theme of feeling present in the supervisee. Some supervisors may not be completely comfortable with Psycards because they are also used as tarot cards. However, it is worth taking a look if you feel the images in these cards will help your supervisory relationship. In online supervision, both parties would need access to the cards.

Issues during a supervisory session

Issues that can occur for some supervisees who are seeing a chronically ill client may be noted during supervision and the supervisor can reflect back what she or he sees occurring. There may be a tendency for collusion to occur with a client because the nurturing side of the supervisee, who can become quite protective towards their clients. It can be quite difficult to know where to draw the line; however, it is important to note that they are a counsellor/clinician and not their client's friend. There will be times when client sessions may be missed due to a client being in hospital; however, one needs to be careful this is not also extended to letting your client miss numerous sessions due to friends visiting, the sunshine, or the need to pick up medication. This can be a delicate balance with a supervisee who feels protective over their client.

Defensiveness is another area that can occur when a supervisee may feel they need to be protective of the client being discussed in supervision. It is quite common to feel that one knows one's client better than the supervisor; therefore, there may need to be some careful discussions so each in the supervisory relationship feels heard. Both parties want what is best for the client in the long run; however, even those clients with chronic illnesses have areas that need discussion.

Some supervisees may have a sense of amazement or wonderment, as termed by Zinker (1977), at how much their client has achieved or succeeded despite having a chronic illness. For some clients, doing as much as possible can distance themselves from the actual feelings they have connected to the illness. A supervisor may reflect on what is actually going on, which can be hard for a supervisee to acknowledge when caught in amazement. Even those who are chronically ill and may have been through many medical battles themselves may not want to encourage an existential crisis from occurring. However, illness can arouse not only the feelings around death for the client but also for the supervisee and supervisor; this can occur not only for those who have a life limiting condition but also those with illnesses that have a normal life expectancy.

Denial, despair, grief, hopelessness, loss, and shock are terms associated with death; however, these also occur with chronic illnesses. The stages of grief and loss depicted by Kübler-Ross (1969) in her book *On Death and Dying* explain a variety of emotions that can occur. Since that publication, organisations such as the Macmillan Cancer Trust have gone further in tending to the needs of those who are ill and dying of cancer. Diabetes UK has a helpline for diabetics who are finding coping with diabetes an emotional struggle. However, there is still a great need for counselling for those with a variety of chronic illnesses. Helplines do assist numbers of people but not in the same way counselling can help. Online counselling is one area that could become a great asset to the NHS, private healthcare or other healthcare organisations across the world.

One reason I believe it is difficult for this need to be seen is that many don't recognise it until they suddenly need it. We are living for much longer periods of time now for a variety of reasons; however, when death does come knocking, people are not usually in perfect health. By putting assistance like emotional support in place for those with chronic illnesses now, we are also giving everybody the capacity to get help when they are older and also need support.

Understanding and misunderstanding

There can be an understanding from the supervisee that the client is living life to the fullest despite having a chronic illness and also see the other areas that the client wishes to discuss. There may also be an understanding that a client may need to attend to their illness during a session. For example, a diabetic client may take a blood test during session or an asthmatic client may use their inhaler which a supervisee may see as normal. It is worth discussing just to make sure there are balanced views on what needs tending to during a session. Supervisees may feel quite uncomfortable, so these discussions can be very useful and psychoeducational. Supervisors can also feel concerned because either they are uncertain about the chronic illness or with conditions they do know about, that they may feel could become life-threatening. A supervisee may have a client with diabetes who blood tests on occasion and the supervisor may have a child of their own with type I diabetes who they have to blood test consistently. In that sort of situation there can be added anxiety for one or both in the supervision session.

Pain disorders are more common than people realise; however, everybody doesn't have the same level of pain because pain is a type of "unknown". In *Body and Psychology*, Kugelmann talks about the management of pain and stated, "Pain, to be pain, must be described" (Stam, 1998, p. 194). If a client says they are using strong medication for pain, for many it may only take the edge off the pain rather than eliminate it. Due to it being an anomaly, each individual tends to assess another person's pain based on the pain they themselves have felt in the past. One person may say the headache they had during a stroke was life shattering and another whose worse injury was falling off a bike may view their pain in the same way; neither one is wrong. For some people, an active day can result in pain for the following day, so they are always balancing what they can and cannot do on any given day. This can be exhausting with chronic conditions so a comment from a client such as, "I feel tired", can have numerous meanings. It can be a fruitful discussion in supervision because each of us will have our own views on the topic.

Much of what I have discussed in this chapter does not really demonstrate that those with chronic illnesses are also having regular lives; they are parents, children, grandparents, teachers, doctors, mountain climbers, scientists, writers, and a multitude of others. Due to many chronic illnesses being unseen, it is hard to tell who has them unless one asks. Even for those with seen chronic illnesses, again, we can only know what they are going through if we ask them. There can be assumptions that all people coping with chronic illnesses have a terrible life, but this couldn't be further from the truth. Only by consulting with our clients can we know what type of life they have and as supervisors it can help to explore with supervisees that discussions with the client are a better option than assuming.

Technology

Technology has moved tenfold in the past few decades and has opened up more avenues of connection and also new are career paths such as online counselling. Due to this, people who live a distance from the counselling centre, or cannot get out freely due to disabilities, can now connect with a counsellor and help to resolve some of their ongoing issues (Jones & Stokes, 2009). Online supervision can take the form of email, message, voice or video via platforms like Skype or VSee; supervision can be one-to-one, in a group, synchronous, and asynchronous (Weitz, 2014). It can happen on an individual basis or as a group, which can be made up of people in different counties or countries. All the creative supervision styles can be used online so any practitioner from any modality can use creativity within their work (Schuck & Wood, 2011).

Technology has also been of great benefit to those with chronic illnesses which have affected their capacity to communicate due to sight, hearing, physical, mental or speech issues. Software such as Dragon has been of great help to those with speech issues or who need the print on the computer to be read out to them. As a result, those with a variety of chronic conditions that were once considered unemployable are getting jobs because they can now communicate. They are also getting counselling because in the past they may have been seen in a medical framework and not necessarily in one where emotional support is at the top of the list.

Technology can also be of assistance to organisations such as the NHS with the limited amounts of room space a GP practice or hospital may have for emotional support. I believe it would be beneficial for GPs to be able to refer their patients to online counsellors, who may see them in less time than presently exists for those needing mental health support. It can be difficult for those needing this kind of support actually to ask for it because there may be a feeling of guilt over the care they may have already received for their medical needs. Some with chronic illnesses also become the "good patient" and feel they shouldn't ask for anything extra. However, meeting one's emotional needs is beneficial for one's medical needs. The body, the mind, and the spirit all exist within a person and each needs varying supports over that person's lifetime. This can be achieved with a teamwork approach where counsellors and psychologists are tending to the mind, medical teams are keeping the body going, and the spirit is also supported by a variety of people. Some of these can happen via online counselling or online medical assistance. Some GP practices now do repeat prescriptions online. The world is changing, and so is the access to health.

Conclusion

In this chapter, I have summarised a number of ways supervisors can work with their supervisees to try to have the best outcome for their clients. Hawkins and Shohet's Process model was mentioned, and I described some creative ways that can be used with supervisees to foster a good working alliance. As my focus was on chronic illness, I also discussed a variety of possibilities and how they can be used to assist the illness with which they have to live with every day. Those with chronic illnesses are now asking for more, and clinicians (for example, opticians, doctors) are now expressing the need for emotional support for their patients. As online counsellors and supervisors, we should be prepared for the diverse range of clients with illnesses who will be requesting our help.

References

Be.macmillan – Coping with and after treatment (2014). Be.macmillan.org.uk. Available online at: https://be.macmillan.org.uk/be/s-592-coping-with-and-after-treatment.aspx.

Ben-Shahar, A. R. (2014). *Touching the Relational Edge: Body Psychotherapy*. London: Karnac.

Bolton, G. (1999). *The Therapeutic Potential of Creative Writing: Writing Myself*. London: Jessica Kingsley.

Cameron, J. (1995). *The Artist's Way: A Course in Discovering and Recovering Your Creative Self*. London: Pan Macmillan.

Chesner, A. & Zografou, L. (2014). *Creative Supervision across Modalities*. London: Jessica Kingsley.

Jones, G. & Stokes, A. (2008). *Online Counselling: A Handbook for Practitioners*. Basingstoke: Palgrave Macmillan.

Jones, J. S., Fitzpatrick, J. & Rogers, V. L (2012). *Psychiatric-Mental Health Nursing: An Interpersonal Approach*. New York: Springer.

Kübler-Ross, E. (1969). *On Death and Dying*. London: Tavistock.

Scaer, R. C. (2007). *The Body Bears the Burden: Trauma, Dissociation, and Disease*. New York: Routledge.

Schuck, C. & Wood, J. (2011). *Inspiring Creative Supervision*. London: Jessica Kingsley.

Freud, S. (1933). *New Introductory Lectures on Psycho-Analysis. S. E., 22*: 1–182. London: Hogarth.

Stam, H. J. (Ed.). (1998). *The Body and Psychology*. London: Sage.

Weitz, P. (Ed.). (2014). *Psychotherapy 2 0: Where Psychotherapy and Technology Meet*. London: Karnac.

World Health Organization. (2014). Global status report on noncommunicable diseases 2014. Chicago: WHO.

Zinker, J. (1977). *Creative Process in Gestalt Therapy*. New York: Vintage.

Chapter 15

The autistic spectrum: its potential impact on online supervision

Liane Collins

First, we will explore autism and what it means to be autistic, then consider its relevance to online supervision, before looking more closely at communication – a core of supervisory practice and main feature of autism.

I'm going to start with an assumption, and that is that anyone either work-ing in counselling or supervision with a neurodiversity issue is going to be very "high functioning" and clients are also likely to be very able to communicate with effectiveness – otherwise the client work would be done face-to-face and most probably in a school or clinical setting. High functioning, of course, is a relative term – and it certainly doesn't mean in every area or all of the time.

Autism

Autism is a specific condition of neurodiversity and culture in its own right in the way in which the world is perceived and experienced. It relates to language and communication, differing abilities, thought processes and attitudes to life, work and daily functioning – and the key feature, sensitivity. People with autism will behave with sensitivity or avoid situations, dependent on their awareness of it, and the physical or psychological senses it provokes. Hyper-sensitivity, of any of the senses, is likely to cause shutdown or meltdown as a defence mechanism.

While there is a core triad of "issues" evident to some degree in each person on the spectrum, their effect and impact varies, as all other features connected with autism also vary greatly, between age, gender, individuals generally – just as they do between anyone else.

Autism tends to be described as a spectrum, but it is a mistake to visualise that spectrum as linear. No-one fits somewhere along a line and stays there. No-one is a little bit or a lot autistic, or high or low functioning, and this idea can lead to making assumptions and stereotyping behaviours. As with most other people, those with autism can change from day to day, with situations, environments or general mood.

Therefore, it may be better imagined as a colour wheel with the primary areas around the outside. Different people will have different strengths and weaknesses in motor skills, perception and sensitivity, executive functioning, social skills, and language and will vary in ability to cope well according to the situation they are in.

When this is shown on a ratio graph, (you might imagine a colour wheel behind it to consider the flow from one area to another), you can see more easily the changes in ability as based on a scale.

The diagram below attempts to explain how some days, in different identified areas, a particular issue may be no problem and other days it is difficult to manage. This particular chart suggests that yesterday the person was feeling comfortable in their environment, able to socialise and talk to people, though had some issues with remembering things and was feeling rather clumsy – perhaps dropping things and getting frustrated. Today however, they really just want to focus completely on one thing – there is a model to build and finish and focus is complete on this task. This means in this case that they are completely unable to give time and effort to communication and socialisation with others. They may also be concentrating so hard because they are feeling hyper-sensitive, or they are avoiding people because of the issue with noise.

More people than ever are receiving a diagnosis of an autistic spectrum condition, and this is now especially prevalent in women as understanding increases as to how autism affects each person differently. The current estimated prevalence is

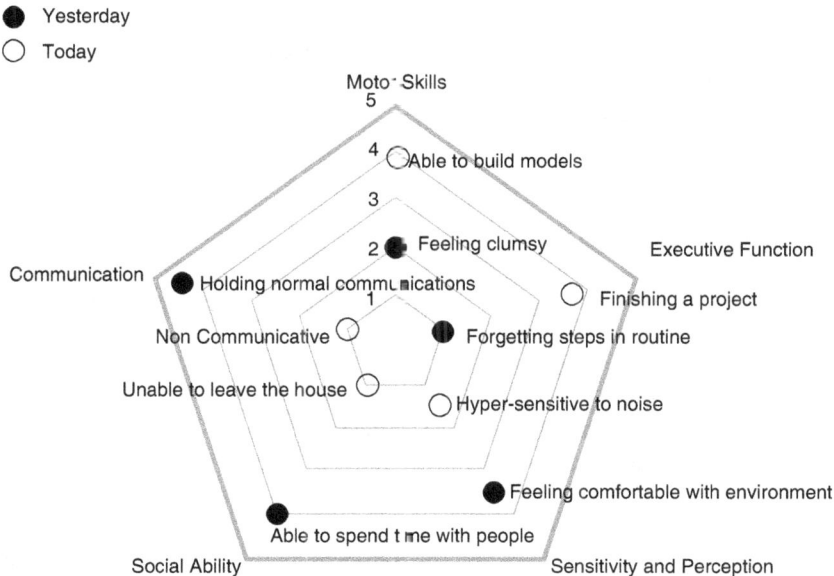

Figure 15.1 Autistic spectrum (Collins, 2016)

one in sixty-eight. In addition, diagnostic criteria have changed dramatically over recent decades. Many autistic people can function successfully in everyday life. With the growth of social media and blogging online, there are opportunities to discuss autism more openly. It may seem as if autism is a huge new thing, but autistic people have always been part of society. Famous historical figures, admired for their work and genius, who are thought by some to be on the autistic spectrum include Albert Einstein, Amadeus Mozart, Sir Isaac Newton, Charles Darwin, Thomas Jefferson, Michelangelo, Hans Christian Andersen, Andy Warhol, and I'm pleased to say a woman made it to that list – the marvellous poet Emily Dickinson.

Supervision

In terms of online supervision, we need to understand the different assumptions and values that influence the behaviour of certain groups. This can be culturally, in all senses of the word. In return, we must also have an understanding of our own assumptions and beliefs. Hawkins (1997, in Hawkins & Shohet, 2012, p. 113) developed a model of five levels of culture, each level influenced by those below.

- ➢ Artefacts – rituals, symbols, art, buildings, policies.
- ➢ Behaviour – patterns of relating and behaving.
- ➢ Mind Sets – ways of seeing the world and framing experience.
- ➢ Emotional Ground – patterns of feeling and the shape making of meaning.
- ➢ Motivational Roots – fundamental aspirations that drive choices.

From the above you may, if you already have any experience of autism, be seeing the pattern.

Autism is significant and unique in the following ways.

- ➢ Rituals and routines, special interests, aloneness, transitional objects, creativity, anxiety, sensitivity.
- ➢ Difficulty in relating to others, varying language ability, rigidity in thinking, avoiding anxiety and conflict, and repetition of actions. Patterns of safety.
- ➢ View of the world – framing experience, differing perceptions and understanding which require exploration in supervision.
- ➢ Coping with emotional extremes, meltdowns, shutdowns, avoidance, hyper and hypo sensitivities, and the avoidance of discomfort.
- ➢ Fundamental aspirations that drive choices – social communication, social interaction, social imagination.

Tyler et al (1991, in Hawkins & Shohet, 2012, p. 114) consider that there are three different ways of responding to difference and diversity. In our specific focus here on autism:

- • The "universalist" would say everyone is different anyway, and possibly everyone has autistic features or that some features are just due to personality.

- The "particularist" would blame everything on the autism.
- The "transcendentalist" appreciates that a person may perceive the world differently but that it is the way in which they move through the world and the choices they make that makes them individual.

As one of the greatest philosophers of our time said: "It is our choices [...] that show what we truly are, far more than our abilities" – Professor Albus Dumbledore to Harry Potter (Rowling, 1998).

We could argue that we are all individuals and so all supervision is cross-cultural, but there is a risk that this could lead to complacency and the "elephant in the room" that is never discussed. Many issues, including autism, are invisible, and are especially hidden online, but may become evident in the ways in which the communication and relationship develop.

Autism is a set of character traits and everyone is different. There can be a high sense of anxiety and shame, so feeling wrong or silly or dumb will push the autistic person into defence mode and shut down to a place of personal safety rather than motivate them.

Hyper-sensitivity can be extremely uncomfortable and so the default position is to avoid or become defensive as a protective mechanism.

Therefore, as supervisors we need to stop, look around, and check out the situation. We need to be mindful in focusing on each sense in turn in detail to bring the experience of the autistic person into the present, rather than being upset about the past and being anxious about the future. This puts you in a much better position to check out what is going on and what to do about it.

Reflective question

What are our own and our culture's idea of a "typical" person with autism?

"If you've met one person with autism – you've met one person with autism!" – Dr Stephen Shore (2013).

A willingness to be open from the start of the relationship offers the opportunity to discuss issues as they arise and how they affect the various relationships.

Based on what we have read, learned from courses, books or others – or our own experience – it can be easy to assume we "know" and understand things. We tend to start within our own frame of reference, and I would argue that there is nothing wrong with this so long as we take a view that allows us to be fluid and permit our experiences of the other person to flow as we gain knowledge and insight into the view from their window. Gentle curiosity and a willingness to learn from each other and about how the other person experiences the world can alleviate misconceptions, blind spots, limitations, and biases.

> ## Reflective question
>
> Are there any accommodations that we feel would be necessary?

Empathy and understanding

The ability to feel is not the same as the ability to express and no one can truly understand another person. Empaths and Autism are not the same thing, though some people with autism are empaths. An empath is so highly sensitive to another person's thoughts and feelings that they know instinctively what those thoughts and feelings are, and may be able to feel them physically. This is contrary to general understanding of autism which assumes that, because empathy and feeling may not be expressed, that it is not felt.

There may also be cognitive empathy, where the thoughts and intentions of others may be predicted, or affective empathy, where the feelings of another can be shared. However, there may be too much empathy and compassion and the emotions can be overwhelming. When there are difficulties with hyper-empathy, it may be necessary to build in self-protection and care, defence mechanisms for self-preservation – perhaps segregating and compartmentalising to organise and cope in stages or at appropriate times. Alternatively, there may be difficulties in understanding other's perceptions, beliefs or emotions. These types of empathy may be constant in an individual, or may change according to the day or the other person.

Few professionals can say what it's like actually to *be* autistic, so paying attention to all our senses online can offer further insight and understanding.

> ## Neurodiversity Facebook forum extract
>
> "Here is my honest opinion; the more I write, read, and talk about autism, the less I know. The less I know makes me curious to learn more. Autism is often just a matter of perception, even some of our most cherished beliefs can change over a few months or years. I see many people trying to own the rights to the autistic spectrum, and yet they can never really do so as everyone's experience is so different. For that reason, I rarely trust someone who says that they are an expert, not that I don't respect them but just that I know they cannot apply what they know to every single person or circumstance. That is why it is good to share experiences, to listen, to learn and most of all, dare I say that word, to be tolerant. We ask for people to be tolerant and yet it we are not ourselves then we are surely becoming what we fear most." Brian

Building relationships

Working online breaks down barriers, making relationships more balanced. There is increasing evidence that real relationships, with warmth and understanding, honesty and congruence, can be built online.

Joyce Thompson and Colin Lago described intercultural relationships in supervision as follows (Stokes, 2011) but adapted to demonstrate how this would appear in a relationship involving autism.

The three triangles offer an opportunity to consider the interaction of supervisor, supervisee, and client, and the client issues, when autism is a feature within the supervisory relationship.

Triangle 1

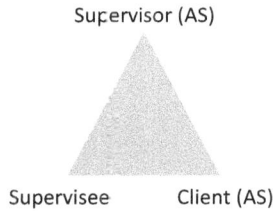

Supervisor (AS)

Supervisee   Client (AS)

Interaction between supervisee and supervisor:

1. The supervisor is collusive with the unseen client.
2. The supervisee has the contact with the client and greater awareness.

Triangle 2

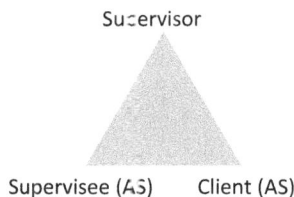

Supervisor

Supervisee (AS)   Client (AS)

Interaction between supervisee and supervisor:

1. The supervisee assumes the supervisor knows little about the issues of both her and her client.
2. The supervisor challenges the supervisee about assumptions made about the client's issues because they share the culture.

Triangle 3

Supervisor

Supervisee   Client (AS)

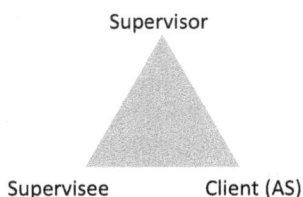

Interaction between supervisee and supervisor:

1. The supervisor and supervisee share a culture and fail to research the impact of this on the client.
2. There is a need to ensure the client is "heard" in their own context. Openness is needed with gentle and genuine curiosity.

Reflective question

What are the implications of this? Blind spots, assumptions, and collusions?

Communication in online supervision

"Sights and sounds are but extraneous noise that clogs the pure expression of mind and soul" – John Suler (2004)

Working online means that it is possible to access counselling and supervision with someone who has specialist knowledge, skills, and experience, even if they are not in your geographical area. This increases the likelihood of cultural difference in some areas, though not in others – such as understanding issues related to disability.

Being online offers balance – a breaking down of barriers. It also may be affected by disinhibition (Suler, 2004), but with sight and sound removed there are opportunities to develop insight from using all our senses and feelings.

Case example

One man who had email counselling said: "I like to write because my thoughts are not in your brain at the same time as they are in mine."

Language can be confusing and difficult to process and it may take a person with autism longer to do this. However, while talking face-to-face can be like trying to speak and translate another language at the same time – then translate it back again for an answer – writing responses is much easier to manage quickly.

Language can also be very vague and be misunderstood. Just because something makes sense in your head, it isn't necessarily what is heard by someone else – autistic or not. It is important when working with people with autism to be careful with language and to be precise.

For autistic people, language may be very formal and time may be taken with longer complete sentences and making sure spelling, grammar, and punctuation are all correct. The way an autistic person communicates may lead to a misunderstanding or misconception of that person.

Many people who work online are asked how they manage without aural, oral or visual cues. This can be beneficial working with autism as often only one sense can be used effectively at any one time – and can be quite intense, shutting out all other sensory cues. Hyper-sensory issues can also often get in the way of effective communication. Imagine having lots of background noise and movement, strange smells and unfamiliar surroundings – then imagine trying to communicate with the person beside you who appears to be talking a different language.

Communication can happen in a variety of ways. Some autistic people think in pictures, and can take a long time to develop fluid spoken language. Some have excellent spoken or written language, but struggle with the unspoken rules of social interaction. Some communicate easily but may not always connect with what is said. Others find alternative methods such as text help them to express thoughts and feelings. In counselling and supervision, despite our first impressions, we must be careful to presume communication competence.

Case example brought by an online supervisee

One partner in a geographically distant relationship was coming for counselling. The couple got on extremely well when writing to each other and texting and had a strong written and online relationship. Unfortunately, things were very different when they were together and they struggled to understand each other in the spoken word relationship. Counselling was sought individually and as a couple to try to work out why this was happening and how they could manage the difficult situation if they continued the relationship as planned and moved in together.

People with autism are assumed not to be able to read body language, but it has been shown that it is not the ability or inability to mirror behaviour or expression that is at fault, but the incongruity perceived from the person performing the action causing reduced social motivation in the person with autism (Hasselmann, 2016).

Reflective question

Would we be afraid to ask questions which might be deemed rude, intrusive or prejudiced – or may not doing so lead to problems later?

Working in online supervision and counselling with autism

Supervision online may allow the supervisee to be more open about their work than f2f. Tricky issues can be explored more easily through "collaborative dialogue" (Anderson, 1997) and "respectful curiosity". The supervisor can validate competence, focus on how the supervisee is working and build on what is going well.

Below, I refer to certain stages of the Page and Wosket (2001) cyclical model for supervision. Chapter three explores this model, the stages of which are contract, focus, space, bridge, and review.

People on the autistic spectrum are often highly visual in their learning. The misconception that there is no imagination is often limited to social interaction. There is often a high ability to identify with stories and characters, so this, with metaphor, simile, and role-play, are helpful ways to investigate, explore, challenge, and also contain both the supervisory and supervisee/client relationships within the supervisory space. This can then be related back via the bridge to the real situation with greater insight and understanding (see chapter three for more detail on the Page and Wosket supervision model, the stages of which are contract, focus, space, bridge, and review)

Creativity can uncover what is happening in the supervisory or the supervisee/client relationships by breaking through meanings and bypassing conscious thought and bringing hidden feelings to the fore.

Autistic strengths in online supervision

➢ Organisation and routine
➢ Highly sensitive – includes intuition, which may be felt physically
➢ May read compulsively and often self-taught
➢ High sense of justice and fairness
➢ Adherence to rules and how the world should work
➢ Adheres to high standards
➢ Difficulties in understanding social hierarchy that tend towards more balanced relationships

Therefore:

> ➢ Promote structure in supervision sessions
> ➢ Make use of self-awareness and exploration in supervision
> ➢ Encourage informative areas and CPD – but also encourage genuine enquiry in client work
> ➢ Build strong boundaries and segregation in relationships – especially important in the dual relationships which occur online
> ➢ Encourage openness and explore assumptions. Encourage to explore difference

People with autism are often highly organised – either because of their love of routine or because they have learned that this is a way to keep anxiety at bay. However, it does mean they will rarely miss an appointment, supervision will be logged and planned to make best use of it, outcomes will be followed up and contracts personally enforced! Some people, because they have hypersensitivities elsewhere, may have developed a sixth sense – insight – or whatever you like to call it. Whatever it is, it may be seen differently, perhaps as pictures and metaphor, or it may be felt physically as a discomfort when something not said needs attention paid to it. Liking to know how things work, people with autism may often read (and buy books) compulsively, spend hours finding things out online and have different pages or books open to follow up threads. The rigidity in the personality works both ways – boundaries are held close and relationships compartmentalised, fairness is very important but expected high standards are also self-induced.

Autistic individuals may:

> ➢ be highly visual and creative
> ➢ relate more strongly to stories and characters within
> ➢ respond well to building and using social stories
> ➢ be unaware or unable to express self when face-to-face
> ➢ have difficulties in visual perception
> ➢ Have alexithymia or other difficulties in expression of emotion

Therefore:

> ➢ Use creativity in the "space" to explore feelings within relationships and alternative scenarios
> ➢ Make use of role-play
> ➢ Try metaphor
> ➢ Use text based communication online – this can create therapeutic distance
> ➢ Be aware that distance can reduce hypersensitivity issues, such as eye contact

- ➤ Try modelling and white boards – drawing lines, shapes and using colour
- ➤ Make use of films and plays – autistic people often watch favourites over and over and relate to their own lives
- ➤ Use music, lyrics, and poetry
- ➤ Use stories and story cards
- ➤ Try letter writing and imagined dialogues
- ➤ Use images and colour to investigate emotions
- ➤ Be aware they may become tired when reading computer screen

Creative online supervision can aid in investigating empathy and the supervisee's feelings towards the client. Role-play can investigate, explore, challenge, and contain the relationship. Working online makes use of therapeutic distance.

Alexithymia is sometimes an issue in autism. It is a personality construct and means that it may be difficult for an autistic person to identify and describe their own emotions, or the emotions of others. The features are a dysfunction in emotional awareness, social attachment and interpersonal relating. This requires effort in building self-awareness and can be greatly helped in supervision with mutual awareness. There may also be difficulties in identifying or naming specific emotions in others, which may be deemed un-empathic or lead to misunderstanding. It doesn't mean there is no awareness of the emotion – just that it cannot be named or explained. Empathy can be greatly felt in AS to a degree where self-awareness and self-preservation are necessary to categorise and contain emotions appropriately. This is also an area for exploration in supervision.

Autistic weaknesses to be aware of in supervision

- ➤ Personal boundaries may be more difficult to hold
- ➤ Often naïve and vulnerable – can be taken advantage of
- ➤ Difficulties in asking for help
- ➤ Emotionally charged or stressful situations may cause anxiety
- ➤ Strong dislike of conflict
- ➤ Social exhaustion and hangover from effort in relationships
- ➤ May have weak short-term memory
- ➤ May struggle to find the right words

Therefore:

- ➤ Take care in use of personal and supervisory contracting
- ➤ Make use of the normative elements of supervision
- ➤ Session contracts and supervision logs can be useful
- ➤ Make use of opportunities for restorative elements of supervision
- ➤ Make use of formative elements of supervision

➤ Promote awareness in supervision and self-awareness
➤ There are advantages to not having to think on feet – there is more time to access reading and research

---

Case example

I had a supervisee ask me what courses could be done or books and articles read to help her and her team understand the increasing numbers of young people who were coming to them for counselling who had been diagnosed or were suspected of being on the autistic spectrum. She said at the moment they were really just listening and counselling on intuition and feeling and making adjustments as they went along. My feeling was that was precisely what they should be doing as they were listening to the individual rather than judging them from what they had learned from a book.

Other issues

Co-morbid issues often go hand in hand with autism, and it is helpful to be aware. In children and young people this may manifest as ADHD and dyspraxia. In adults, it is likely to be depression and anxiety issues. Research indicates people on the autistic spectrum may be far more likely to have an associated condition, and so may also be diagnosed with:

➤ Gastrointestinal disorders
➤ Sensory problems
➤ Seizures and epilepsy
➤ Intellectual disabilities
➤ Fragile X syndrome
➤ ADHD
➤ Bipolar disorder
➤ Obsessive Compulsive Disorder
➤ Tourette's syndrome
➤ General Anxiety Disorder
➤ Tuberous sclerosis
➤ Clinical depression
➤ Visual problems
➤ Hearing problems
➤ Dyspraxia
　(www.autism-help.org/index.htm)

However, it can be difficult to determine if these are associated issues or part of the autism itself.

Mental health issues may increase the risk of suicide ideation and many of those admitted to hospital may also have autistic features, though I have found no research evidence to back this. In terms of online supervision, it is worth being aware that a supervisee with a diagnosed or suspected autistic client may be more likely to be working with higher risk, not only of intent but as someone who may also not share their intention to self-harm or carry out suicide.

While rules are stuck to rigidly, including boundaries in contracting, personal boundaries can be difficult to hold. There are risks of taking on too much when there is a desire to be liked or helpful, or strong personal feelings of guilt when asked for help. A first instinct may be to pull back from a need to "fix" a difficult situation.

An awareness of difference and appearing difficult can make for wariness in asking for help in the autistic person – either not noticing or not admitting to difficulties until it is too late, considering that issues might not be of interest to anyone else, or an unwillingness to "put on" to someone else.

With a strong dislike of conflict, working online provides the distance to cope with more challenge in the work. Challenge and constructive feedback can often be taken personally. While synchronous work offers the potential to deal with the fallout immediately, working asynchronously gives opportunities to work through different scenarios, thoughts and feelings before responding.

Hypersensitivity to emotion can cause extra anxiety which is difficult to work through and understand and then discharge. This, and the extra effort required to communicate and cope with relationships, can cause exhaustion and hangover.

There may be short term memory issues – though long term is often not a problem!

Finding the right words, especially when under pressure or emotionally charged, can be difficult and can cause stuttering or mutism, which is less of an issue when working online.

Sometimes learning is a bit slower. Sometimes people with autism just want to make sure they have it right before they show the world they can walk! But the more you know and understand the easier it is. The autistic brain is just wired a little differently. This makes some things more challenging but also an interesting experience.

Awareness can be helpful in supervisory sessions and coping strategies understood and put into place. We also need to remain aware that difference does not need to be corrected to suit our own view.

In the words of Albert Einstein (1952): "I have no special talents. I am only passionately curious."

Reflective questions

What "truths" or myths did you already know about the autistic spectrum?

What would you like to know more about related to AS and other diversity issues?

What will you take away with you from this to inform your online practice in diversity and/or wit⁻ AS?

Does your knowledge about specific issues of difference and diversity impact on practice?

References

Anderson, H. (1997). *Conversation, Language, and Possibilities: A Post-Modern Approach to Therapy*. New York: Basic Books.

Einstein, A. (1952). Letter to Carl Seelig. *Einstein Archives, 39–013*.

Hasselmann, H. (2016). No, autistic people do not have a "broken" mirror neuron system – new evidence. BPS. Bps.org.uk. Available online at: www.bps.org.uk/content/no-autistic-people-do-not-have-broken-mirror-neuron-system-%E2%80%93%C2%A0new-evidence.

Hawkins, P. & Shohet, R. (2012). *Supervision in the Helping Professions (4th edn)*. Berkshire: Open University Press.

Page, S. & Wosket, V. (2001). *Supervising the Counsellor: A Cyclical Model (2nd edn)*. London: Routledge.

Rowling, J. K. (1998). *Harry Potter and the Chamber of Secrets*. London: Bloomsbury.

Shore, S. (2013). *Countdown to the Conference: What Will Speaker Dr. Stephen Shore Say?* Available online at: www.autismspeaks.org/blog/2013/06/27/countdown-conference-what-will-speaker-dr-stephen-shore-say.

Stokes, A. (2011). Cross-cultural supervision. *TILT Magazine – Therapeutic Innovations in Light of Technology, 7*: 62–64. Available online at: https://issuu.com/onlinetherapy institute/docs/tiltiss7.

Suler, J. (2004). The Online Disinhibition Effect. *Cyberpsychology and Behavior, 7(3)*: 321–325.

Further resources

Ashton Smith, J. (2011). *Autism Spectrum Disorder and Girls*. Middletown: Centre for Autism. Available online at: www.middletownautism.com/fs/doc/publications/mca-booklet-0004-wlink.pdf.

Burgess, R. (2016). Comic redesigns the autism spectrum to crush stereotypes. Available online at: https://themighty.com/2016/05/rebecca-burgess-comic-redesigns-the-autism-spectrum/.

Marshall, T. (2014). Moving Towards a Female Profile: The Unique Characteristics", Abilities and Talents of Young Girls with Asperger Syndrome. Available online at: http://taniaannmarshall.wordpress.com/2013/03/22/moving-towards-a-female-profile-the-unique-characteristics-abilities-and-talents-of-young-girls-with-asperger-syndrome/

Further learning

www.autism.org.uk
www.autism-help.org

http://autismmythbusters.com/general-public/famous-autistic-people
http://elearning.autismwestmidlands.org.uk/store
www.rainbowautism.org
www.autismmatters.org.uk
www.autangel.org.uk

Chapter 16

Supervising online: couples counselling

Stephanie Palin

Introduction

In this chapter, I will be exploring the complex work of relationship counselling, and the ethical and confidentiality issues that may arise in supervision in this specific area of counselling. I will be using casework examples which have been anonymised to protect the confidentiality of clients in line with *BACP Ethical Framework for the Counselling Professions* (2016).

The modes of online working that will be considered are email, instant messaging, and web cam counselling, each of which brings both similar and different issues in respect of working with couples.

Relationship counselling

Relationship counselling is a term used to describe counselling provided for adult couples who have, or have the capacity for, a sexually intimate relationship, and is preferred to the term "marital counselling" which is more frequently used in the USA. The term relationship encompasses a wide variety of couple relationships – gay, straight, cohabiting, civil partnered, married, or couples living separately but who see themselves as an intimate couple. Relationship counselling may involve the couple together or just one partner. In email counselling and instant messaging, it is more common for the counselling to involve one of the partners, although the other partner may be encouraged to use the medium too. It is not possible to invite a partner to engage in the counselling process without first obtaining permission from the client partner for reasons of confidentiality.

There may be a variety of reasons why one partner may seek help without telling their significant other, and whilst this is not encouraged, it is the client's choice as to whether they involve their partner, or even tell them that are having counselling help. It could be that one partner does not accept that they need help, whilst the other is aware of the difficulties they are experiencing and has been unable to resolve them without external help. There are also couples in which one of them holds the belief that they "should not air their dirty linen in public – it should be kept within the family". This can lead to further resentment between the couple and become an additional source of problems.

Relationship counselling is offered to one partner using the systemic concept that change in one family member will affect the whole system, and that the client is the couple relationship (Bobes & Rothman, 2002).

Couples often present for counselling when their communication has broken down to the extent that they are unable to resolve the issues that they have without outside help. For some couples, their communication has never been good, with their interactions based on assumptions and their past experience. In most cases, greater clarity in communicating with openness and transparency leads to a better understanding of themselves, their partner and their relationship. However, for others, their relationship survives because they do *not* communicate in any depth, and encouraging them to do so may disrupt the balance that they have achieved as a working model for them. Such couples are often successful individuals who have an active social life involving friends and family, but who rarely spend time alone as a couple. Generally speaking, however, most couple counsellors would agree that the best outcome for couple counselling is that the couple become more self-aware, more aware of their partner, and more knowledgeable about their couple relationship, which allows them to be able to grow and change together.

Although the couple are the experts in their relationship (Anderson & Goolishan, 1992), the counsellor is the one who can guide them through the conversations that will help them make better sense of it. One of the key things that couples with problems do, is to triangulate a third party into their relationship. The third party can be a person, issue, substance, child or any entity that takes the focus off the relationship and thereby reduces the tension. This is one of the key concepts of Murray Bowen's theory (Bowen, 1978; Kerr & Bowen, 1988). Whether working face-to-face or through an online medium, the counsellor may become the triangulated person who reduces tension for the couple. This may result in a couple who become dependent on the counsellor and counselling to maintain an equilibrium in their relationship. "Many couples protect themselves against excessive intimacy by avoiding every opportunity of attaining a strictly one to one relationship" (Willi, 1982). The therapeutic relationship itself may become an emotionally intimate one when couples are willing to be honest and open and to share their developing self-awareness, and for some couples, this then presents a dilemma of which they may be only dimly aware. They may act out their discomfort with the intimacy of the therapeutic relationship by cancelling sessions, asking to meet less frequently, or simply by disappearing from therapy. Whether working face-to-face or online, it is important that clients are clear about what contact, if any, the counsellor has with clients between sessions, and what contact it is acceptable for clients to have with their counsellor. It is also true, as Knox and Cooper (2015) state that "some clients are not ready or able to relate at depth" (p. 87). They go on to observe that sometimes a lack of deep connectedness can be just as useful as relating at depth.

Systemic therapy is a valuable theoretical base from which to formulate questions that promote change, and also encourages the counsellor to take a collaborative, non-pathologising position with the clients (Bobes & Rothman, 2002). Circular and reflexive questions encourage clients to consider new meanings to their experience of one another. As Karl Tomm (1987, p. 172) writes:

> Reflexive questions are questions asked with the intent to facilitate self-healing in an individual or family by activating the reflexivity among meanings within pre-existing belief systems that enable family members to generate or generalise constructive patterns of cognition and behaviour on their own.

Sometimes, in email counselling, I will suggest posing a series of questions at the end of the therapeutic reply as a stimulus to reflexive thinking. Asking questions is best done in an invitational way, so that clients do not feel interrogated. For example, "you might want to think whether…" or "I wonder whether you have considered…". I also suggest: "You might like to consider these questions, and let me know what thoughts you have had about them in your next email."

A supervisee, Jenny, had done this with Tom and Julie, a couple who had presented with a lack of sex in their marriage. Jenny's encouraged them to send weekly emails, but they sent one per month which led me to the hypothesis (Cecchin, 1987) that they had problems with emotional intimacy which had caused the problems with physical intimacy. When Jenny sent the exploratory questions, she received no response at all.

Six months later, she received a reply from Tom and Julie – a bullet pointed list headed: "Answers to your questions".

They did not include the list of original questions, and no further dialogue; just the answers to the questions. It was as though the clients were engaging with the work, but at a very limited level. As Jenny worked with this couple, she found them difficult to connect with, and we became more certain that my hypothesis about their avoidance of emotional intimacy was correct.

Analysis of her therapeutic replies to the couple in supervision helped Jenny to see that she had approached the work in her usual warm, empathic way, but that this may not have been enough for Tom and Julie as they struggled with intimacy, both physical and emotional. One of the central tensions that couples struggle with is that of balancing intimacy, identity, and independence. For example, an individual may question whether they can retain their identity and still be part of a couple relationship, or whether they will "lose themselves" in the relationship. Another person may believe that when they get close to someone, they lose them, so in order to feel safe, they maintain distance, both emotionally and physically.

The online disinhibition effect (Suler, 2004) means that some clients disclose more frequently, more quickly and more intensely than they would face-to-face and this in itself may result in a client's defences coming into play as their unconscious fears of intimacy determine their willingness to continue with therapy. They may withdraw to a more superficial level of relating, leaving the counsellor wondering what has happened to the developing therapeutic relationship, or they may leave therapy, often without warning. It is always worth considering whether the client's choice of medium for counselling has been based on their avoidance of intimacy.

On the other hand, when working with email therapy, clients may become immersed in the intensity of the relationship and respond immediately to a therapeutic email in their desire to maintain connection without having time to reflect on the content. This may lead a client to become overwhelmed by the intensity of the process and of their own emotions, without a supportive enough environment to contain those emotions. Most online counsellors build in a time lapse between receiving an email and responding to it therapeutically. There are several reasons for doing that, but amongst them is to help the client read, digest, and reflect upon the issues discussed before penning reply. Many counsellors regulate the time interval by building that into their contract with clients –for example, suggesting weekly exchanges of email, or that they will respond on a specific day of the week. A time lapse also enables counsellors to get supervision help on a dilemma without delaying the response to the client.

When working with counsellors new to working in text, I offer to review their reply to clients before sending to the client. This gives a safety net as a new counsellor may miss something important, or say something that could be misinterpreted by the client. In general, after six to ten emails, their work does not need further scrutiny.

The number of words that a client sends to a counsellor will also vary enormously, and it often helps to give a suggested word count to the client of, say, five to seven hundred words initially. Whilst some clients find this constraining (especially the client who sent an initial email that was 12,768 words long), others find that it focusses them on what they really think the problem is, and what help they require. I list some questions that they might like to think about in composing their email, and some clients find them helpful (below). In doing this filtering, they are thinking about their relationship and will already have begun the process of counselling.

- Why are you seeking help now?
- When did the difficulty start?
- What did you notice?
- Who else is involved or affected by the problem?
- What have you tried so far to manage the situation?
- What goal(s) are you aiming for as a result of this counselling?

Jenny and I discussed Sandra, the "client of the 12,768 words" in supervision as Jenny had felt overwhelmed by the length of the email, which had included many email exchanges between Sandra and her husband David over a period of four years. Jenny had reviewed her contract for counselling that she sent out prior to starting work and realised that she had not been clear about the five-to-seven-hundred-word limit. She had given it as a *suggested length*, rather than a maximum limit. One way to avoid this dilemma is to have a form for the client to complete that only allows seven hundred words. However, I have known clients who have got around that by writing without spaces between words, so that the whole appeared to be one word, and was incredibly difficult to read! Having a limit on the number of characters avoids that.

Jenny did state in her contract that she allocated an hour to responding to an email, and so was able to say to Sandra that it would take longer than an hour to read and digest what she had written. Jenny suggested to Sandra that she would read what had been written, but that Sandra then needed to edit it down to seven hundred words describing the problem and what she was seeking from counselling, and that Jenny would then reply to the edited version. Whilst Sandra was initially unhappy about that, she went ahead, and she worked with Jenny for two years, ending with Sandra leaving her abusive husband safely. An analysis of transcripts of face-to-face sessions of an hour's length by Day and Schneider (2002) found there to be a mean of just under six thousand words, whereas an online session of the same duration produced a mean of just under two thousand words. My usual practice is to respond to the client with around 1,000–1,200 words, allowing time to think and to reflect as well as write, and this is what I suggest to supervisees.

Sexual difficulties are presented online more frequently than face-to-face and this is understandable as many people find it difficult to talk about sex, even with their intimate partner –or particularly with them. Despite the proliferation of sexual information available online, many clients with sexual problems do not access it. Magazines have many articles about sexual performance and having "hot sex" but this may leave a couple with sexual problems feeling isolated, and that they are the only people with a problem. All too often the sexual problem is, and remains, the "elephant in the room" as far as the couple is concerned.

Being able to explore the sexual problem by email, or live chat means that the client does not have to make visual contact with the therapist. Even if they later switch to webcam counselling, the therapeutic relationship has usually developed to such an extent that the problem can be talked about. This is not always the case, however, and I worked with a couple where loss of desire on the man's part was their issue, and the female partner never appeared on screen. I had ten sessions with the couple, but only heard her disembodied voice, whilst he was in camera for the whole time. She wanted to have input to the sessions and was willing to be involved in the sex therapy, but did not want to see me or have me see her. This was a strange experience, but what I picked up from her voice was her anger towards her partner, that he currently did not want to have sex with her. Like many women, she perceived her husband's loss of desire as a reflection on her sexual attractiveness, thinking that he would "fancy her" and want to make love to her if she was desirable. There are, of course, many reasons why a person loses desire, sometimes just for their partner and sometimes more globally.

When sex therapy is undertaken with a client couple, it is advantageous to work using web cam, so that feedback can be obtained from each partner about the set tasks they have undertaken at home during the preceding week. The therapist often has to tease out the answers to their questions about how the task went and by email this can become a somewhat drawn out process which is unhelpful to the counselling.

I worked with a couple in France who were both academics. He was from England and this was his first live-in relationship at the age of forty-two, whilst she was a very sexually experienced American woman of thirty-nine who had moved into his apartment when the lease ran out on hers. I was initially, working via email – his chosen medium – on his erectile problems. After their first series of tasks (three-hour long sessions of a sensual touching exercise with both partners naked), I asked for feedback, giving them some prompt questions. I received a four-page document from her outlining how the exercises had gone in her view, with each session clearly delineated. His response was: "It went well. I enjoyed it."

After supervision, I decided to ask them to use web cam, which they agreed to. When they both appeared on camera, she sat at least a foot in front of him, partly obscuring him from the picture. He was as reticent in this medium as he had been on paper, and each time, I had to ask him very direct questions to elicit his reactions to the tasks. He was initially very uncomfortable and felt intimidated by her experience and sexual demands. She also made it clear that asking her to abstain from sexual activity whilst they learnt new and beneficial ways of interacting intimately was totally unacceptable and not possible for her. I was on the receiving end of her anger, just as he was. Whilst some progress was made over several months when they both committed to the work, therapy ended when she was offered a prestigious academic post in Norway and he encouraged her to accept it. I could see his relief when she announced that she had taken the post and would be moving on.

Case study

A female client connected via web cam. She was having an affair and wanted help to decide whether to leave her controlling husband. She described her lover as her soulmate, and said she had never felt so loved and alive. It was through this relationship that she realised how much her husband controlled her life and how unhappy she had been, despite their affluent lifestyle.

Her dilemma was whether to leave this very comfortable lifestyle. Her children were being privately educated at eminent boarding schools, and they had homes in the country, central London, Switzerland, and the Mediterranean. She spent her days gardening, shopping, and organising a couple of charity balls per year. The wellbeing of her children was also very important to her.

I was struck by her secrecy in setting up the webcam sessions. Although we usually spoke from her home, she used different rooms, even once being in the guest cottage. There were sessions from her mother's house, the Swiss ski lodge and even the garden of the Mediterranean property whilst everyone in the family was in bed – this latter held in whispers.

In one particular session, held in her home, we discussed what might need to change in her marriage for her to continue to live with her husband. Since she had owned how

hard it was to think about losing her lifestyle, I wondered whether she might be able to make changes that would make her happier, even if it meant giving up her lover. The session appeared to go well, so I was surprised when I got an email from her three hours later stating that something really urgent had come up – could we meet again that afternoon?

This was highly unusual, and demonstrates how easily clients can make contact with us, even when boundaries about the limits of contact have been set.

I agreed to the session as this usually unflappable client was clearly upset by something.

Apparently, her behaviour in disappearing off with her laptop had raised her husband's suspicions that something was "going on", and he had recorded her session with me. He had then returned home and confronted her about it.

This led me to wonder:

- To whom the recording belonged,
- Whether he had acted illegally in recording the two of us without permission,
- What I would add to my contract with clients about recording sessions,
- What more I needed to say to clients about holding responsibility for their online safety and confidentiality.

Supervision of relationship therapy online

Instant messaging

Most instant messaging sessions are conducted with one partner from the relationship, and when both partners participate, it is helpful for the counsellor to be able to distinguish which client is writing. With systems such as Skype chat it is easy to see who is writing and who is watching, but some of the systems such as Moxie, used by Relate, only have one space for the client to type in. In such systems, it is helpful to ask the clients to preface what they write with their initial, so that it is clear to the counsellor which partner is speaking. It is a good exercise for couples who struggle to give each other space and who find it hard to listen to each other. When one of them is typing, the other has no choice but to wait and read until their partner has finished, particularly if they are sharing a computer and keyboard. It might be the only time that they really listen to what their partner is saying. It is sometimes a good idea to suggest that they spend time communicating in this way – or by email between sessions, until they are able to really listen to and value the partner's views.

The advantage of instant messaging is that a full transcript can be used in supervision, so that an analysis of interventions and a discussion of the underlying intention on the part of the counsellor can be discussed in depth. A discussion of the theories and the nuances of the words used by both client and counsellor can yield valuable learning. Of course, consideration must be given as to how the transcripts are stored, and how they are transmitted to the supervisor for supervision. In private practice, it is prudent to hold as little client material as possible on the counsellor's computer, with transcripts and emails transferred to an external hard drive which can be locked away securely. Organisations who deliver Live Chats will have secure servers where the transcripts are held.

For many years I have supervised counsellors in Relate where many of the instant messaging sessions are one – off sessions from clients in crisis with their relationship and it is important to form an instant rapport with the client. Once the client feels that the counsellor understands their situation, they are willing to engage and open up. It is acknowledged that the client often wants help in managing the difficulty that they have presented. To assist in thinking about what is helpful, I have developed a model for this type of work as shown in below.

The Equss Model

E   empathy
Q   questions
U   understanding
S   specific
S   suggestions

Inexperienced counsellors often go straight to asking questions, which can leave the client feeling interrogated rather than understood, so stressing the empathic connection right from the start is invaluable. I have found, on many occasions, that when clients have said that the session has not helped them, examination of the transcript shows that the counsellor has failed to express their *empathy* in words. An intervention such as: "You really are having a tough time aren't you?"

or "Goodness, you are juggling such a lot!" is often enough. To go through a transcript line by line and look at where an empathic comment could have been inserted is a valuable exercise for counsellors who struggle with this area. A counsellor may feel anxious to be helpful or to know more, and get drawn into asking questions. I cannot emphasise enough how important the expression of empathy is. When working with a client face-to-face, a counsellor's empathy is expressed in a number of ways, some verbal, some non-verbal. A smile, a frown or other facial expressions can show that you understand what they are saying or how they are feeling, and these need to happen through words in this medium and in email.

Asking *questions* is the next step in order to find out what is going on, and the first one is usually "how can I help you today?" and after the client has outlined their issues, "Which of those things do you want to talk about today?"

Reflexive questions will help the client clarify and *understand* or see their situation from a different perspective – sometimes seeing their partner's view of the situation by asking a question such as, "and if your partner was writing to me, how would they describe your present dilemma?" Such questions aid their understanding of why they are not feeling heard or understood or why their partner is resisting listening.

And the final step is to make *specific suggestions* which might be for them to speak with their partner, or to read a webpage that is sent — or to seek further counselling, maybe with their partner, by webcam. The suggestions are always couched in tentative terms as something the client might like to think about. Using this model in supervision, in conjunction with a transcript of a session, enables a counsellor to see what they might do differently as well as affirming their good practice.

Email counselling

Supervision of email counselling is often done online by email or web cam. In writing about their casework, it often happens that the counsellor gains insight or clarity simply from writing about their relationship with the client and the relationship problems they are working with. The email the counsellor sends often has the same effect on the counsellor as it has on the client –the situation becomes clearer, and a way forward offers itself. Of course, care must be taken in sending any client material, and a form of encryption is recommended. The very least that needs to happen is that any identifying names or details should be removed, and the document password protected. Each counsellor uses their own password, and I reply with a further password. As stated before, I hold both client material and supervision on an external hard drive which can be locked away, and nothing is retained on my laptop or desktop.

If both partners are involved in the counselling, an agreement needs to be made as to how they will communicate with the counsellor. Sometimes each partner contributes to a joint email, and the counsellor replies to both of them. If the clients are sending separate emails to the counsellor, it is essential to agree with both partners whether the material is to be confidential or can be shared in part or whole. Generally speaking, individual emails are confidential between the client and counsellor, so when each partner is writing separately, specific agreement needs to be made with each of them about sharing what is written. If the clients want their individual emails to be kept confidential, the counsellor may be left with information that the partner is not aware of, for example that an affair is ongoing, or that one partner is thinking of leaving. Once the counsellor knows the secret, they are placed in a difficult position. If they hold the secret, then they are colluding with the partner with the secret, and at some stage, if the secret emerges, the other partner may want to know whether the counsellor had been aware of it. If a secret is told to the counsellor, then it is for the counsellor to discuss in supervision whether it is something that will interfere with the counselling process. If, for example, a client had not told their partner about a life event before they met, it may be that the incident could remain unknown to the partner. Clients are encouraged to share things with their partner, but there are occasions when they feel unable to do that, and the counsellor judges that counselling will be possible without it being known. This needs to be revisited if it becomes apparent that the previous event *is* having an effect on the work.

I insist that counsellors consult in supervision where domestic violence and abuse (DVA) is presented or even hinted at, so that we can discuss the circumstances and offer the most appropriate way forward. It is important to consider whether distance counselling might put the client at greater risk. Helping to ensure that the client is safe and has a plan to stay safe is valuable work, but couple counselling is rarely advisable other than face-to-face.

Because emails are asynchronous, that is they do not take place in real time as a live chat does, both counsellor and client have more time for reflection between communications. Most counsellors who use email allow a minimum of two days in which to respond. This needs to be clear in the contract made with the client at the start of counselling, so that their anxiety does not rise as they wait for a reply. This has become more important as the use of the internet has advanced. The use of social media such as WhatsApp and Instagram means that more people are used to instant responses when they communicate something via the internet. There may also be times when a client's mental health means that they are not able to tolerate time gaps between their email send and the counsellor's reply.

One of the areas of ethical concern is a client's mental health and their capacity to use email as a medium for therapy.

Case study

A supervisee, Jack, had begun email counselling with Charlene whose marriage had ended because of her husband's serial affairs. Jack made a very clear written contract for weekly email exchanges and that any contact between those exchanges would be for administrative reasons only. After a few sessions, Charlene said that she could only afford sessions fortnightly, and Jack replied to say that he believed that she needed more support than that, and if she could not afford to work with him on a weekly basis (she was already being offered a heavily discounted rate), he suggested that she might need more frequent support and that perhaps she could access help through her doctor. He added that he would continue to work with her until she could source such help. This elicited a stream of several hundred emails at all hours angrily accusing Jack of abandoning her. In supervision, we explored possible reasons for this surprising development. The main theory that we worked with was that of transference, which was once thought of as a concept relating predominately to psychoanalytic therapy, but which now is conceptualised in a way that embraces many therapies. Flaskas (2002, p. 139) states that:

> Within contemporary thinking, transference is used more to describe the process of a person recreating his or her patterns of emotional experience in the context of the current analytic relationship. Transference, then, is about an individual's pattern of relating.

As we explored what was known about this client, there was a pattern of bombarding people to whom the client had been close with attempts at contact when the other person had created distance. This suggested an attachment style that Bartholomew, Henderson, and Dutton (2001) describe as preoccupied. Such a person longs for close relationships, but does not believe that they are lovable and when a relationship ends, they are likely to pursue the other person and show emotional dysregulation. Pursuing someone is all too easy to do online and their lack of responsiveness is perceived as abandonment. Jack and I decided that he would email Charlene, offering to help her to access support via the NHS, and that he would work with her again when she was more able to use counselling effectively (by this point, he was aware that Charlene had previously been under the care of the mental health team). In addition, he said that he would not respond to any emails or texts, but that if she went for three months without contacting him at all, Jack would contact her in order to ask whether she still wanted counselling with him. Whilst this was a drastic action, it set boundaries for the therapeutic relationship.

It is clear that working online with relationships provides different ethical considerations from one-to-one work, and a different dynamic. Couples may well reach the desired outcome of better understanding of themselves, their partners and their relationship together, but it is also possible that they become embroiled in conflict with the counsellor as observer to that. It is important that, whatever the counselling medium, the counsellor is robust in their responses and has courage in their interactions (Bond, 2016). As Anthony and Nagel (2010, p. 136) state:

> The BACP guidelines make a point of highlighting that practitioners should be aware of the additional complexities of working with couples in this way and ensure that they are properly trained and prepared for it.

References

Anderson, H. & Goolishian, H., (1992). The client is the expert: A not-knowing approach to therapy. In: S. McNamee & K. J. Gergen (Eds.), *Therapy as Social Construction*. London: Sage, pp. 25–39.

Anthony, K. & Nagel, D. M. (2010). *Therapy Online: A Practical Guide*. London: Sage.

Bond, T. (2016). *Ethical Framework for the Counselling Professions*. Lutterworth: BACP.

Bond, T. (2009). *Ethical Framework for Good Practice in Counselling and Psychotherapy*. Lutterworth: BACP.

Bartholomew, K., Henderson, A., & Dutton, D. (2001). Insecure attachment and abusive intimate relationships. In: C. Clulow (Ed.), *Adult Attachment and Couple Psychotherapy: The "Secure Base" in Practice and Research* (pp. 43–61). Hove: Routledge.

Bobes, T. & Rothman, B. (2002). *Doing Couple Therapy: Integrating Theory into Practice*. London: Norton.

Bowen, M. (1978). *Family Therapy in Clinical Practice*. Northvale: Aronson.

Cecchin, G. (1987). Hypothesizing, circularity, and neutrality re-visited: An invitation to curiosity. *Family Process, 26(4)*: 405–415.

Day, S. X. & Schneider, P. L. (2002). Psychotherapy using distance technology: A comparison of face-to-face, video, and audio treatment. *Journal of Counseling Psychology, 49(4)*: 499–503.

Flaskas, C. (2002). *Family Therapy Beyond Postmodernism: Practice Challenges Theory*. Hove: Brunner-Routledge.

Kerr, M. & Bowen, M. (1988). *Family Evaluation*. New York: Norton.

Knox, R. & Cooper, M. (2015). *The Therapeutic Relationship in Counselling and Psychotherapy*. London: Sage.

Tomm, K. (1987). Interventive interviewing: Part II. Reflexive questioning as a means to enable self-healing. *Family Process, 26(2)*: 167–183.

Suler, J. (2004). Online disinhibition effect. *Cyberpsychology & Behaviour, 7(3)*: 321–326.

Tomm, K. (1988). Interventive interviewing: Part III intending to ask lineal, circular, strategic or reflexive questions? *Family Process, 27*: 1–11.

Willi, J. (1982). *Couples in Collusion: The Unconscious Dimension in Partner Relationships*. Claremont: Hunter House

Chapter 17

Supervising online counsellors of young people

Jan Stiff

Background

Recently trained in online counselling, and having experience of counselling young people face-to-face, I began working for an online organisation that offered online counselling to young clients. My first client was a young person who shared how she had regular suicidal thoughts. These thoughts later developed into a fully formed definitive suicide plan.

After a number of online counselling sessions, I reached a critical point where I felt as if I could have readily given up on my client. I felt desperate. Empathy was turning to frustration, anger, and fear. The sense of risk began to feel overwhelming. I was becoming immune to the meaning of the word "suicide". It was likely that I was reaching a stage of burnout.

However, I was lucky. My supervisor showed care and understanding. I felt safe and able to express my fears openly. She shared invaluable skills, experience, and knowledge in counselling young clients in an online environment. Importantly, I trusted her and did not feel judged.

My online supervisor helped me reflect, learn and develop from this experience. She was invaluable to my being able to continue counselling this client safely and effectively.

A personal interpretation

The provision of online counselling for young people is an expanding area but this is occurring at a time where there is a scarcity of supervisors specifically trained in online supervision and an even greater scarcity of practitioners with experience and skills in supervising online counsellors working with children and young people (CYP).

Counsellors working with children and young people online need to have an understanding of the lives and development of young clients, with particular understanding of mental health and mental illness in this age group along with their online behaviours. Colleagues providing supervision to these counsellors need to have an equal, or better, understanding in order to provide appropriate support, challenge and development.

This chapter aims to provide an introduction and brief overview of the role of the online supervisor offering supervision to counsellors counselling young people online. Much information originates from insights and experience acquired during personal practice and study. It is not intended to provide formal guidelines for practice or definitive answers. Instead, this chapter aims to enable the reader to consider elements that they find helpful as a start to expanding their knowledge or practice. Since every young client, every online supervisee and every online supervisor are unique, some points within this chapter are likely to be up for discussion and I would welcome readers' feedback. Please note that as the subject of safeguarding is referred to only briefly within this chapter, it is important to acknowledge its significance in the field of online CYP counselling and subsequent supervision. Unfortunately, I am too restricted by space within this chapter to be able to explore this subject and related issues, to their totality – It would require a chapter in itself. Chapter ten also addresses some of these.

Introduction

There are a number of significant differences between counselling young people online and counselling adults online. These can be attributed to differences in lifestyles, emotional, physical, and intellectual development and behaviours, as well as issues around mental health and available support and treatment for this age group. The first part of this chapter therefore begins by providing a broad account of the typical world of a young person, followed by an indication of the differences between online counselling and face-to-face counselling within this age group, challenges faced by online counsellors, a comment on the issue of vicarious trauma and a comment on issues surrounding counselling of children and young people in the UK.

The second part of this chapter proposes a model for online supervisors' work that provides a flexible framework for online supervision, whilst incorporating these differences and reflecting upon the value of the relationship between the online supervisee and online supervisor.

The term "online (CYP) supervisee" will be used for counsellors counselling children and young people online. The term children and young people can be taken to include adolescents from about the ages from eleven to twenty-one years. "Online supervisor" will be used for supervisors providing supervision for online (CYP) supervisees, and implies a knowledge and skill in counselling children and young people online in their own right.

Part one: the young person's world

Figure 17.1 illustrates typical elements of many young people's lives. They live in a multifaceted and complex world, over which they have very little control. It makes sense that during this time, they commonly share how they feel pressurised, isolated, and misunderstood. These commonplace pressures are complicated

"Lures and Pitfalls-

The Darker Side of Adolescence"

- Alcohol abuse
- Dangerous trends
- Drug abuse
- Extreme risk taking
- Gambling
- Gangs / Groups / Cults – the need to belong / gain identity
- Sexually transmitted diseases
- Social media – e.g. online grooming, sexting
- Underage sex / teenage pregnancy
- Violence

Broken line denotes weak / dysfunctional or abusive relationship

Full line denotes strong / supportive relationship

Regular "Pressures and Challenges"

- Body image
- Bullying
- Coping with physical and or learing disabilities
- Desire for independence from family
- Desire to feel safe and nurtured
- Deteriorating mental health services
- Economic status
- Emotional development
- Enjoying living on the edge
- Family support / isolation
- Feeling misunderstood
- Grief and Trauma
- Hormonal changes
- Mental "ill Health"
- Peer pressure
- Physical development
- Prejudices
- Relationships
- Risk taking
- School / Further Education - Study
- Physical / Sexual / cultural identity
- Social media / Media

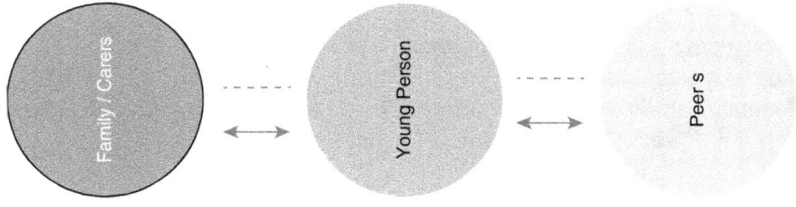

Family / Carers

Young Person

Peers

Figure 17.1 The young person's world

further if a young person lacks a supportive and nurturing environment and background and essential elements required for building resilience.

Within this diagram, the young person takes the central place. His or her family/carers and peer group are a predominant influence and may or may not have a positive influence upon the young person (indicated by a broken or full line).

It is important to understand the role of peers in a young person's life – hence their equal presence alongside the family/carers. "Successful peer relations, positively contribute to the development of social skills and feelings of personal competence that are essential for adult functioning" (Ingersoll, 1989 cited in Wolfe & Mash, 2006).

Skills knowledge and attitudes required of an online (CYP) counsellor and supervisor

I suggest it is fundamental that both practitioners have a firm, basic knowledge of the following:

- Attachment theory/attachment disorders
- Effect and significance of peer relationships
- Effects and significance of family dynamics
- Effects and significance of school life
- Development of the adolescent brain
- Importance of boundaries
- Mental health disorders, for example, low self- esteem, anxiety, depression, self -harm, eating disorders, suicidal thoughts
- Rights of young people
- Significance of loss and change within a young person's life
- Transference and countertransference online
- Young people with disabilities/physical and learning. For example, the autistic spectrum disorder (ASD) since online counselling can be more effective for young people with ASD. For instance, there is less sensory overload. A valuable comment came from a discussion with Liane Collins, a fellow contributor specialising in Asperger and Autism conditions, said in a private conversation:
  "It is more important to listen and be willing and able to adapt according to the view of the world held by their client."
- Young people and the law
- Young people who might present as particularly vulnerable/isolated/misunderstood, e.g., gender dysphoria, children in care and those termed NEET (not in education, employment or training)
  ("Understanding where adolescents have come from developmentally and their needs as emerging young adults is essential if the supervisor is to be of use to the counsellor", Henderson 2006).

A number of these factors might be frequently changing or shifting for a young person, intensifying any feelings of vulnerability or fear.

It is important for the online (CYP) counsellor and online supervisor to ensure their knowledge base is up to date (e.g., any changes in the law). I would like to suggest that suitable, up to date knowledge of these factors make up a significant part of an online (CYP) supervisee's and online supervisor's "tool kit"– this way they are prepared for any issues that might arise within an online (CYP) supervision session. It is important not to forget another integral part of an online supervisor's tool kit – feedback gained from one's own senses or "gut feelings" during a session. These will have been gained from experience and knowledge that might not be accessible in the moment, as well as transference and counter-transference encountered within a session. If your antennae are attuned to these and they are managed well, this "unconscious stuff" can be the one of the most valuable aspects of online CYP supervision.

Reflective question

Stoltenberg and Delworth (1994) in Page and Wosket (2013) propose the following developmental stages of counsellor supervision:

- Level 1 – "Highly motivated, anxious, and dependent upon the supervisor [...]"
- Level 2 – "Motivation fluctuates. Moves between autonomy and dependence upon the supervisor [...]"
- Level 3 – "Increased sense of personal counsellor identity, autonomy, and professional self-confidence [...]"
- Level 3 Integrated – "A level not achieved by all. Therapist becomes fully functioning counsellor or 'master' practitioner"

Reflecting on these stages, and applying them to online (CYP) supervisees, which stages in an online (CYP) counsellor's development do you feel you would be able to confidently provide online supervision for?

Young people online – challenges for the online (CYP) counsellor

A report by Rawson and Maidement (2011) identified the following issues encountered by counsellors counselling young people online. These can be related to young people's online communication within a session and, in my experience, can also occur during online supervision sessions, usually with countertransference as the root cause:

- Lack of verbal and visual cues – imagination and fantasy become a possibility.
- Anonymity and identity – who is the young person communicating with? Is it a person, powerful adult, computer screen? Few online counselling organisations offer totally anonymity for their young clients. Alongside that, there is always the possibility that a young client could provide incorrect personal details.
- Asynchronous thoughtfulness – any saved communication can be read at a later date and reflected upon or shared with another person outside of the therapeutic relationship.
- Depth and immediacy of disclosure – young people make disclosures of high levels of distress more quickly and more commonly online than face- to-face.

In my experience, the following are often discussed within online supervision and relate back to Rawson and Maidement's report (2011). These issues can be a source of much anxiety for the supervisee, before, during and after an online (CYP) counselling session. (Please note, these are not in order of significance.)

- Assessment of young person prior to online counselling (For example, assessment of competence/ability to make informed decisions online, anonymity or detailed contact information, agreement of confidentiality, contracting) – "How can this be done effectively? How detailed does it need to be? Will it affect the beginning of the therapeutic relationship?"
- Lack of endings – "The black hole effect" – Suler (1997). There is no assurance that there will be a response or maintenance of communication from a young person during an online session. Likewise, there is no certainty that they will return to the next, booked, session. To this effect, each message/ counselling email, needs to be managed as if it could be the last contact. The online (CYP) supervisee might ask/ assume: "Why? Is this my fault?" through to; "Have they died by suicide?"
- Online disinhibition – Since a young person might feel they are confiding in a "computer" rather than a sensitive, human being, and while not having to make eye contact, they may be less guarded in their communications. For instance, issues of anger and frustration might be more openly displayed towards the counsellor. A lack of "netiquette" might leave the young client perceived as being "curt" or "rude".
  "They say things to us because we're not in the room and they don't have to deal with our expressions" (Sefi, 2011).
- Managing disclosures – organisations offering online counselling for young people will have an appointed safeguarding officer. However, it is the online counsellor who the young person communicates with in the moment. The online counsellor is often required to make an assessment and management decision during the session or immediately afterwards. This assessment and

decision making requires specific knowledge, experience and skilful communication. In some instances, online counsellors question their ability to attend to the counselling process where they are frequently attending to safeguarding issues. In a discussion with Lalage Harries, a specialist in the field of safeguarding young people online, and a contributor to this book, she offered the following valuable and reassuring advice:

"When counselling young people, if you're not attending to risk, you will not be able to do anything valuable therapeutically."

- Transference and countertransference – either may or may not be recognised by the online counsellor during or after an online session. The skill of the online supervisor and relationship between both counsellor and supervisor are essential to help manage this issue. The effects of transference and countertransference can be particularly powerful when working with young people online – for this reason, the supervisor needs to be attentive to the restorative side of supervision (Proctor, 1986) and recognise that this can be a frequent and significant part of the supervisory process when supervising online (CYP) supervisees. This is a particular issue that can be usefully discussed and explored within the supervisor's own online supervision of supervision.
- Being "in the moment" – online platforms can be easily accessed via mobile phones. Since young people usually have their mobiles readily available, online counselling can be accessed at the acute moment of their distress.
- Misunderstandings – an issue that can unquestionably be encountered during online counselling, requiring close vigilance and caution from the online counsellor. For instance, caution needs to be paid to the use of irony and humour online. Either can be misinterpreted and understood as offensive if used inappropriately.
- Boundaries within the online relationship – it is my experience that online counsellors frequently find it more challenging to maintain boundaries with a young person who decides to break or challenge them in an online session, when compared to face-to-face counselling.
- Perceived power within the online relationship – how do the young person and online counsellor relate to each other? Misguided perception of the other can lead to an imbalance of power in the relationship. In reality, this might be unintentional or intentional.
- The counsellor's own story – identifying with a young person might be more powerful for those who are able to reflect on difficulties within their own history as an adolescent. Online disinhibition contributes to the influence of this sensation: "Through projective identification, the therapist may get an unbearable feeling of what it is like to be that child" (Pattison, Robson, & Beynon 2014).
- How can I be "me"? – online counsellors with relatively little online experience often struggle with how they can be "real" online and build a rapport with a young client. Reflecting on their ability to counsel a young person face-to-face is often helpful.

- Working with risk – The decision to "hold, share, or report" – each decision can result in distinct feelings of discomfort and bring powerful emotions for the online supervisee (CYP) These can feel more intense due to the effects of online disinhibition from the young client, powerful transference and counter-transference: "Supervisees can bring complex and overwhelming feelings to supervision, issues of counter-transference may be at work or real-time sympathy and despair for a vulnerable child" (Pattison, Robson, & Beynon 2014).
- Young people and their mental health – mental health, mental health issues, mental health disorders, mental illness – what do these terms mean to the young person, their online counsellor and the online supervisor?
- Knowledge of common pharmacology – used in young people's mental health.
- Technological problems – to avoid disruption in the online supervisory process, preparation for potential problems and knowledge of common technological issues are essential.
- Knowledge of routes for referral, locally and/or nationally as appropriate.

These challenges illustrate the skills and knowledge required to provide an understanding of the young person, and how they typically communicate and behave online. This, in turn, requires skilful management within the online (CYP) counselling relationship. If an online (CYP) counsellor is well informed and prepared, it helps to ensure the young client maintains their trust, allowing the therapeutic relationship to continue and develop. These challenges will inevitably have some effect upon the online counsellor and will form the background for the thoughts, reflections and issues they bring to online supervision. Of particular interest to me is the issue of "vicarious trauma".

Vicarious trauma

Within my own practice, I have encountered moments where online supervisees have shared emotions and behaviours (e.g., encountering regular, intrusive thoughts about their young client) which are likely consequences of vicarious trauma. It does not seem to be uncommon within online (CYP) counselling sessions, confirming why this subject merits singular focus within this chapter.

> It is our belief that all therapists working with trauma survivors will experience lasting alterations in their cognitive schemas, having a significant impact on the therapist's feelings, relationships and life. (McCann & Pearlman, 1990)

Understanding the powerful influences that online disinhibition, online transference and counter-transference can have upon the online (CYP) counsellor, vicarious trauma is more likely to occur within this line of practice when compared to face-to-face counselling (CYP).

Online disinhibition often allows young clients to be explicit in their communications with an online counsellor and, online counsellors working in this field, are more frequently providing counselling for distressed and suicidal young clients. Research published by Evans (2014) stated:

> The young people [...] indicated that they prefer the online environment when discussing their suicidal ideation and that in cyberspace they have found a space where they feel safe to discuss their turmoil in complete confidence.

Etherington (2000) writes expansively on this subject in an article for the *British Journal of Guidance & Counselling*. Though she writes about vicarious traumatisation through counselling victims of sexual abuse, much of what she writes is appropriate here. Etherington offers the following as reasons for complex counter-transference:

1. Identification with the victim
2. Identification with the role of rescuer
3. Identification with the abuser

Etherington also suggests the following for supervisors supervising counsellors presenting with vicarious trauma. To attend to:

1. Balanced workload
2. Protective strategies
3. The impact of the context: "[...] trauma can be exacerbated and repeated within organisational contexts [...]"
4. Modelling good boundaries
5. Finding meaning in experience
6. Remind ourselves why we do this work

If an online (CYP) supervisee feels they have been affected through vicarious traumatisation, or if our discussion reflects this as a possibility, I would gently discuss the significance of investing time for some personal therapy in order to protect themselves and their young client. This is where the relationship between an online supervisor and their online supervisee (CYP) is key, and where supervisors need to be careful not to let their role become unintentionally blurred with that of a counsellor.

The present state of online counselling for young people – an escalating challenge

> It is time for us all to recognise that most young people will seek information online first to deal with their emotional and mental health difficulties. (Balick, 2013)

Experts are now recognising this is a specialist field requiring that counsellors have specific knowledge, expertise and skills relating to mental health issues of this age group. Likewise, I would suggest that their online supervisors require the same level of knowledge, and expertise, if not more, in order to support their online supervisees soundly.

Balick (2013) says:

> [...] a combination of intense concern about self-harming and powerful discomfort in discussing it, is sending young people online in droves seeking answers.

Childline's annual review for 2015/2016 stated that more than two thirds of their counselling sessions take place online. The top three issues that children and young people presented with were "low self-esteem/unhappiness, family relationships, and bullying/online bullying". However, at the other end of the scale, the charity reflects the increasing number of counselling sessions for suicidal thoughts, this being at its highest ever levels.

Many young people continue to access online counselling for concerns around bullying, family, and relationship issues. During a discussion with Stephanie Palin, a consultant at Relate, online trainer, and contributor to this book, she informed me of the following relating to her practice:

> By far the commonest problems brought to the work are relationship ones: Relationships with parents, teen age boundary issues, plus the impact of separation and divorce and also relationships with stepparents, at school – bullying and friendships.

Within my private practice as an online supervisor of online counsellors (CYP) I have also noticed an increase in more complex and severe mental health issues presenting within supervision sessions. It is likely that continuing NHS funding pressures have a large influence to bear.

The organisation Young Minds (2016) reported on the increased waiting times for CAMHS (Child and adolescent mental health services) and the effect this is now having: "Without treatment, children are more likely to self-harm or become suicidal, to be violent and aggressive [...]."

For both online supervisees (CYP) and their online supervisors, it is important to have a good knowledge of the common mental health issues affecting young people and how these might be divulged during online counselling. I would suggest that these "common mental health issues" can include disclosures of self-harm and suicidal thoughts, dependent on assessment.

Part two: a proposed model for online supervisors supervising online counsellors (CYP)

At present, there are no published models specific to online supervision or online supervision for online (CYP) counsellors.

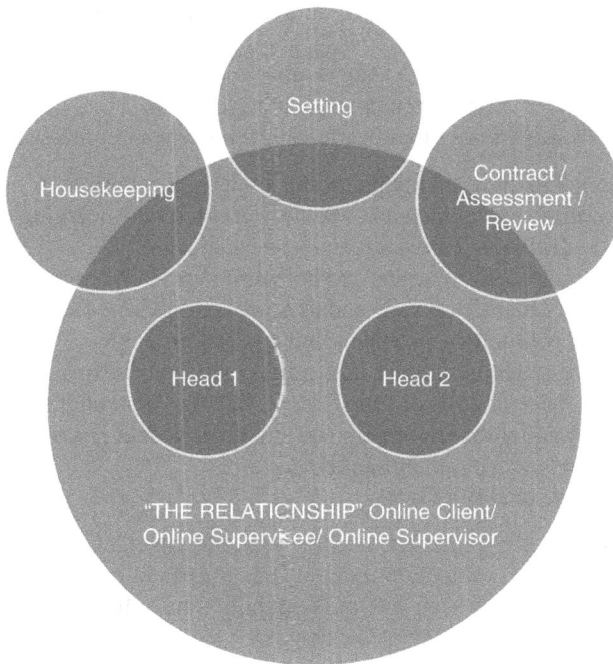

Figure 17.2 The face of online supervision (CYP)

Basing the requirements of an online supervisor on what has been previously written in this chapter, the aim of this model is to provide a simple framework or checklist for navigating the variety of skills required of an online supervisor to ensure safe and effective practice. It is hoped that the simplicity of this model makes it memorable whilst paying attention to significant elements of this field of online supervision and the importance of the relationship between the online supervisor and online (CYP) supervisee.

The following model echoes aspects of three models that have inspired my practice and were chosen because they are transferable to supervising (CYP) online. It is suitable for use in both private and organisational settings.

1. The three functions of supervision (Kadushin, 1985; Proctor, 1986 in Carroll, 2012):

    •   Educative (formative)
    •   Supportive (restorative)
    •   Administrative (normative)

    The Formative or "educational" aspect of supervision is a vital element since the field of young people's mental health, safeguarding and the law relevant to young people online are frequently changing fields, requiring the online supervisor (CYP) regularly attends to regular continuing professional development.

2. Hawkins and Shohet (2012) offer a more comprehensive list of the elements of supervision called the "primary foci of supervision". This provides a regular space for the supervisees to reflect upon the content and process of their work.

- To develop understanding and skills within the work
- To receive information and another perspective concerning one's work
- To receive both content and process feedback
- To be validated and supported both as a person and as a worker
- To ensure that as a person and as a worker one is not left to carry unnecessarily difficulties, problems and projections alone
- To have space to explore and express personal distress, re-stimulation, transference or counter-transference that may be brought up by the work
- To plan and utilise their personal and professional resources better
- To be pro-active rather than re-active
- To ensure quality of work

3. The third model is a medical model proposed by Neighbour (2010). Though not a new model, it inspired much of this proposed model, particularly the "housekeeping" element – one of Neighbour's five checkpoints. (The others are connecting, summarising, handing over, and safety netting).

"The face of online supervision (CYP)"

This model reflects the online supervisory needs of online (CYP) counsellors and the importance of working in a relational way whilst providing a framework that is flexible, allowing me to work with the therapeutic approaches of online (CYP) supervisees.

Working relationally, I aim to build a rapport with an online (CYP) supervisee that expresses care, respect, and trust whilst acknowledging them as an individual, with individual experiences and lives. "The respect for difference forms is an integral part of the negotiating process between two people in any communication" (Gilbert & Evans 2000).

At a time where safeguarding issues appear to be an escalating focus within online counselling sessions with young people, the quality of the relationship is key to provide a space in which the online supervisee (CYP) feels safe and emotionally "held" whilst they express and explore situations in their practice that might have left them feeling helpless, ashamed, guilty or fearful.

Reflective questions

- What is your view about using models in online supervisory practice?
- What would you require from a model to help you in your practice?

Viewing this model simply, it is not dissimilar to a face with two eyes and something not too dissimilar to curly hair, hence the name – "The face of online supervision". It is a simple diagram, and easy to remember visually.

Two "heads" within a "head"

The central, large, circle is where the relationship between the young client and the (CYP) supervisee lies. This is the focus of online (CYP) supervision sessions acknowledging that successful supervision relies on a good therapeutic relationship between the online (CYP) supervisee and their online supervisor.

Within this central circle are the two heads. I have adopted these from Neighbour's model (2010), originally designed for general practitioners' (no apology is being made for being influenced by this model. I and others have been influenced by Hawkins' and Shohet's "process model" (2012), initially intended for the helping professionals but now strongly influencing the field of counselling supervision).

Neighbour (2010) names the two heads as the "organiser" and the "responder". He explains how each "head" will take it in turns to be in charge. This echoes just how my thoughts function during online supervision sessions where the young person is at the heart of the session. On reflection, I realise that I continually operate in anticipation of the fact that a safeguarding issue regarding a young person might be brought to my attention or that I might need to highlight a safeguarding concern with my supervisee. These two "heads" are similar to two antennae; for me they are continuously attentive and almost, instinctive throughout a session.

For me, the "organiser" is the critical, analytical, organised, and informative part of my thought process and practice. Most importantly, it helps to ensure that online supervision remains safe and ethical.

The "organiser" is similar to Schön's process of "reflection-in-action" (cited in Rikard, 2011): the internal supervisor within a therapy session.

Neighbour (2010) describes the second head as the "responder" – it is " [...] an altogether more spontaneous and naïve part of you [...] the responder is intuitive. It notices everything uncritically"

The "responder" is described as being affected by all the senses and tunes in to what is being communicated verbally and non-verbally – it pieces all these messages together and notes the emotions and feelings resulting from them. In the absence of visual and verbal cues when working online, the "responder" could help in recognising and managing transference.

Reflective questions

- Do you feel you need to/or pay enough, attention to the "organiser and responder heads" within sessions with an online (CYP) supervisee?
- How could the "organiser and responder heads" aid you in your practice?

The two heads are at the heart of the supervision process. They work together as a constant, and allow me to pay attention to the relational side of supervision – to concentrate and reflect upon transference and countertransference made possible from the relationship that I have with my online supervisee and the relationship that they, in turn, have with their young online client.

There are three smaller circles that lie along the top of the central circle as they are essential for providing good supervision. In some sessions, I might pay minimal attention to one or more of these circles, for example, when the focus of the session requires attention to the supportive needs of the supervisee. They all merge with the central circle. Even if my "organiser" head pays minimal attention to them, they are always present, ready to be brought to the forefront of my attention at any time, ensuring that I work ethically and professionally.

Circle 1: "contract, assessment, and review"

I have taken this from the cyclical model by Page and Wosket (2011) inspired by the elements of "review" and "contract" and combined them. This is an essential part to any online, supervisory relationship. This contract may not be mentioned in each supervision session but it influences all aspects of the session. It ensures it is boundaried and helps to ensure that I work in harmony with my supervisee. For example, since online supervision can be vulnerable to technical problems, all contracts made with my online supervisees have alternative contact details and a plan in the eventuality of technological failure. It helps us feel more secure should an issue occur. Making space for reviews and assessments helps to keep both myself and my supervisee informed of our progress and any need to attend to our learning updates.

Reflective question

You are formatting a contract for a new supervisee. They work for an organisation that provides online counselling to children and young people. You also have a second, new supervisee, who works in private practice providing online counselling for young people aged twelve years and above.

Considering both circumstances, what significant differences will there be between the contracts you propose for each online counsellor?

Circle 2: "setting"

This is adapted this from the Hawkins and Shohet "seven-eyed model of supervision" (2012, pp. 86–88).

It is, simply, the setting within which the supervisee is working and accountable, and the setting within which I am working and accountable, or controversially it might be where I am working in private practice. It is important to bear in mind how it affects my practice and how it requires managing. This might be beneficial or counterproductive. For instance, when providing online supervision for a counsellor working within an organisation, the policies and guidelines of that organisation need to be taken into account – or in some cases, they might need reviewing from reflections made in an online supervision setting. I need to agree to/or ask for clarification concerning these policies and guidelines from the beginning as they inform my work with the online (CYP) supervisee.

Circle 3: "housekeeping"

For me this aspect is vital: "housekeeping" comes from Neighbour's (2010) *The Inner Consultation*. Neighbour (2010. p. 87) states, "housekeeping" is "concerned with stress prevention", which I feel is a vital component of online (CYP) supervision.

I see this as the time before, after and in-between online supervision sessions. Hawkins and Shohet (2012, p. 122) explain how, in the helping professions, "[...] we can be caught up in a negative cycle of stress, making us less effective, which leads to further stress".

The main issue within housekeeping is the self- recognition of stress and the steps taken to deal with it. Personally, online supervision of my online supervision practice is the most significant part of "housekeeping" in an effort to prevent and manage stress and ensuring I am suitably challenged on my practice.

Scenario

You reach the end of a particularly stressful session with your online (CYP) supervisee: Your computer went offline once during the session and there were moments where there was a delay between messages.
Reflecting on the purpose of the three circles;

- How could you have prepared for any technological problems?
- What other options were available to you when your computer went offline?
- How can you address potential computer issues within the contract between yourself and your online (CYP) supervisee?
- What do you need to include in the contract to ensure that your online (CYP) supervisee is also prepared for possible technological issues from their computer (either personal or organisational)?

Meeting the needs of the Online (CYP) counsellor and the young person, through online supervision

Table 17.1 illustrates how this model can be used to focus on particular issues relevant to supervising supervisees who counsel young people online. For example, significant elements or issues, such as online disinhibition and online safety, are acknowledged a number of times within the model highlighting their importance.

Conclusion

To conclude: (CYP) Counselling online requires a different set of skills and attributes from f2f work. Supervising (CYP) counsellors requires a firm understanding of specific, and often unique, issues and skills in order to be effective and useful. There have been few answers or conclusions made within this chapter. That is for the reader; the online (CYP) counsellor, endeavouring to understand what they might require from an online supervisor; the supervisor who wishes to expand

Table 17.1 Illustrating the "significant elements" present within this model

Significant Elements	Head 1	Head 2	Contract, Assessment, Review	Setting	Housekeeping
Mental Health Issues	X	X			
Restorative Supervision		X			X
Online Disinhibition	X	X		X	
Assessment	X		X		
Boundaries	X			X	
Online Safety	X		X	X	X
Integrative, Relational approach	X	X	X		
Therapeutic Practice of Supervisee	X		X		
Private or Organisational Setting	X		X	X	
Normative Function	X		X	X	X
Formative Function	X		X		X
Restorative function		X	X		X

their work into the field of supervising online (CYP) counsellors; or the online supervisor already in practice who wishes to ensure that their continuing professional development is up to date and that their practice is adequate.

I am passionate about online (CYP) supervision and I am going to bravely state that, if we have an interest in young people and desire to enter into this specialist field of supervision, we owe it to ourselves, our online supervisees and their young clients, to commit to regular supervision of our supervision, making it a priority in our work.

> We know from neuroscience that a practitioner can be simultaneously flooded with the same, unhealthy cortisol as is the child they are listening to [...]. The supervisee needs a containing supervisor to increase her own opioids and diminish cortisol. So, too, the supervisor has to hear the pain and contain splitting, and he or she needs to keep up their own regular supervision of supervision for identical reasons. (Pattison, Robson, & Beynon 2012)

References

Bailick, A. (2013). Online support strategy needed. Youngminds.org.uk. Available online at: www.youngminds.org.uk/news/blog/1238_online_support_strategy_needed.

Carroll, M. (2012). *Counselling Supervision – Theory Skills and Practice*. London: Sage.

Childline (2016). *Annual Review 2015–2016 – It Turned Out Someone Did Care*. Available online at: www.nspcc.org.uk/globalassets/documents/annual-reports/childline-annual-review-2015-16.pdf.

Evans, S. (2014). A thematic analysis of preferences of young people using online support to discuss suicide ideation. *International Journal of Transactional Analysis Research, 5(1)*.

Etherington, K. (2000). Supervising counsellors who work with survivors of childhood sexual abuse. *Counselling Psychology Quarterly, 13*: 187–190.

Gilbert, M. C. & Evans, K. (2000). *Psychotherapy Supervision: An Integrated Relational Approach to Psychotherapy Supervision*. Buckingham: Open University Press.

Hawkins, P. & Shohet, R. (2012). *Supervision in The Helping Professions (4th edn)*. Buckingham: Open University Press.

Henderson, P. (2006). Supervising work with adolescents. *Therapy Today, 17*.

MacKay, D. (2016). Waiting times having devastating effect on vulnerable children. Youngminds.org.uk. Available online at: www.youngminds.org.uk/news/blog/3390_waiting_times_having_devastating_effect_on_vulnerable_children.

McCann, I. L. & Pearlman, L. A. (1990). Vicarious traumatization: A framework for understanding the psychological effects of working with victims. *Journal of Traumatic Stress, 3*: 131–149.

Neighbour, R. (2010). *The Inner Consultation – How to Develop an Effective and Intuitive Consulting Style (2nd edn)*. Oxford: Radcliffe.

Page, S. & Wosket, V. (2011). *Supervising the Counsellor: A Cyclical Model (2nd edn)*. London: Routledge.

Pattison, S., Robson, M., & Beynon, A. (Eds.). (2014). *The Handbook of Counselling Children & Young People*. London: Sage.

Proctor, B. (1986) Supervision: A cooperative exercise in accountability. In: M. Marker, & M. Payne, (Eds.), *Enabling and Ensuring*. Leicester: Leicester National Youth Bureau and Council for Education and Training.

Rawson, S. & Maidment, J. (2011). Email counselling with young people in Australia: A research report. *Women in Welfare Education, 10:* 14–28.

Rickard, A. (2011). The internal supervisor. *Therapy Today, 22*: 26–29.

Sefi, A. (2011). Online counselling for young people. *Therapy Today, 22*.

Suler, J. (1997). The black hole of cyberspace. In: *The Psychology of Cyberspace*. Available online at: http://truecenterpublishing.com/psycyber/blackhole.html

Wolfe, D. A. & Mash, E. J. (Eds.) (2006). *Behavioural and Emotional Disorders in Adolescents: Nature, Assessment, and Treatment*. Abingdon: Guilford Press.

Chapter 18

Online supervision in a university setting

Kirstie Adamson

Online supervision in a university setting

Universities are times of transition. Students attending university, at whatever age, are engaging in a change in their lives. Achieving a degree will, they hope, enable them to get a job, change career, or establish a long-held ambition. It is also the first time that the majority of students have left home and face independence. Universities are also short term. Unless you are proposing a university career then the aim is not to stay at university. This makes it very different from other stages of life later on. For this reason, issues often arise in a university setting which have not done previously. In this chapter, I hope to address the issues that seem to arise more often in a university setting. I am not proposing to look at all issues that arise as those will be well dealt with in other chapters.

Online supervision – how it takes place in a university

When online counselling happens in a university it is usually a small part of the workload of the counsellor. Supervision may be provided by the university or the practitioner is required by the university to have appropriate supervision whether this is paid for by the university or by the individual practitioner according to their contract.

The reality is that most counsellors have face-to-face supervision with supervisors who have little or no knowledge of online counselling as most of their work is face-to-face. Counsellors usually do not want to have two supervisors.

Whose responsibility is it to ensure that supervision is appropriate for online counselling?

According to *BACP Ethical Guidelines*, it is the responsibility of the counsellor to ensure they have adequate supervision. It is usually the counsellor who dictates how long the supervision will be for and what clients are brought to supervision. When online counselling is a small part of the work load of a counsellor, it may be that the interests of the university are best served by providing online supervision.

How does this take place? It is a question I have pondered. Initially when I first set up online counselling at the university that I work in, I had a good online supervisor and quickly took a certificate in online supervision to enable me to provide the supervision for my colleagues.

BACP recommend that supervision is separate from line management. So, this was potentially an issue when later on I also had some line management responsibilities. However, all our counsellors have independent external supervision and the additional online supervision did not preclude this. On the basis that the online supervision was for any issues particularly pertaining to online counselling and each counsellor would in addition be able to take their client to independent supervision, it felt okay.

This was fine when my supervisor worked nearby and I could have a mixture of online and face-to-face supervision. But when my supervisor started her process of retiring and stopped working nearby, it meant that all my supervision suddenly became either by telephone or online. I missed the face-to-face work and despite the amount of online work I did, the majority of my work was still face-to-face. Universities rarely support a practitioner to have two supervisees and so I was stuck in a cleft stick. Either, my online clients and my online colleagues were well provided for and I had online supervision, or my face-to-face work was prioritised and I had no support with online work. I could not manage this ethically. I needed to re-think things.

Practically it can be an issue to comply with this BACP requirement as there are often restrictions on what supervision can be accessed within any organisation. I spoke to other universities to find out what they did to meet that requirement.

A different way of providing supervision online and complying with this part of the ethical guidelines is to provide peer supervision for each other. It still has its problems because practitioners who are not as experienced in online counselling as others will inevitably feel less confident in providing supervision. There are five counsellors at my university all with differing experiences in online counselling. Clients are allocated according to availability but some counsellors have had more online clients than others. We are now operating a pool of peer supervision to each other when we have online work. If I have a query that feels bigger than our level of expertise within our group then we will seek out a one-off supervision with an external online supervisor. But peer online supervision is working well.

Encryption

The Supplementary Guidance Working Online by BACP (2015) states that, "Good practice safeguards [...] includes adequate password protection and encryption of services being provided" (p. 6). It is important therefore that universities only offer online services appropriate to their security. Not all universities offer SMS counselling for this reason and stick with email asynchronous counselling. This is good practice. The same applies for supervision.

Confidentiality

Confidentiality is discussed more fully in chapter ten on legal and ethical implications. As in other agencies, there may be greater need for disclosure than when working privately. These might be for professional suitability, fitness to study or conduct. Each university will have its own guidelines for managing this but it needs to be really clear in any contract. Usually this is all accounted for within a Privacy or Confidentiality statement.

Data Protection Act 1988 and General Data Protection Guidelines 2016

A university counselling service is more likely to receive requests for copies of client notes DPA and shortly GDPR than in private practice. This can be for any number of reasons but mostly because either a client wants to see and keep a copy of their notes or because the client has gone to the police about a crime, e.g., past or present abuse or assault. The police will often want to have copies of the actual notes despite offers of a brief report. They may also wish to interview the person concerned even if that person has left the university.

Without consent of the client there is no legal compulsion to disclose notes to the police unless there is a production order from the Court. In my experience, most requests from the police come accompanied by a request from the client.

If a client is receiving online counselling, then the whole session will be available. It is also likely that the client will have all the notes themselves. What is important to remember however, is if there is online supervision then the notes of that will also be in their entirety and may need to be made available on a request for disclosure. This is only relevant if there is supervision within the service internally. Therefore, clear guidelines about how long the notes will be kept for are essential. The Data Protection Act 1998 states that notes should be kept for a reasonable time. How long this might be for is up to the service. It may well be for a shorter time than the notes kept on the actual counselling. However, notes can be redacted. This means that anything relating to a third party (in this case the counsellor) can be crossed through with a black line (see chapter ten on legal and ethical implications).

Universities have clear guidelines for how counselling notes are kept. It is important that equally robust and clear guidelines are made for keeping supervision notes. These need to be kept separate from client notes however.

Risk

What is appropriate within a university setting for online counselling and what is not?
How do supervisors assess this with their supervisees?
When does the risk involved feel intolerable for the university?

Establishing guidelines about what feels appropriate for the university that you work in is essential. There is no rule about this as long as the counsellors are clear. Some universities will not work with suicidal ideation online, others will. My sense is that a client is potentially safer interacting with a counsellor than with no one, so unless it becomes clearly dangerous and external referrals are necessary

I would advocate working with a client. The guidelines that I have worked under are that online counselling will no longer be appropriate when:

1. The client has insufficient English to manage online communication.
2. When a client is suicidal and has other activation that makes it unsafe, e.g., a client who is actively suicidal and at the same time hearing voices was deemed not appropriate for online counselling.
3. When the client does not use the counselling appropriately, e.g., the client consistently finds fault with the counsellor in a way that starts to feel like bullying? This can be very subtle so that the counsellor begins to dread the emails she receives.

This should be the clinical decision of the counsellor with the support of the online supervisor, subject to the guidelines operating at your university.

My concern remains – what happens if you stop online counselling and ask the client to make direct contact and then the client then stops accessing help at all?

In email counselling N is writing more and more about his sexual activities and wishes, having always felt previously that he could not talk about sexual matters. Talking in this way would have been forbidden according to the culture he lived in, both in his family and his religion. The counsellor is feeling uncomfortable as if she is being asked to be a voyeur. There is a concern that he could be using the counselling for sexual excitement rather than to deal with the issues.

But what happens if when the counsellor invites N in for a face-to-face session he does not mention the sexual activation he was describing in online counselling? Some clients will bring up totally different issues online from face-to-face. This then becomes an area for supervision. Online counselling may have provided the only safe space to talk about sexual issues. It is extremely difficult for clients of some cultures to work with sexual issues and online counselling can be an area that makes it feel safer. The tightrope decision is whether this is therapeutic or being used inappropriately.

Helen reported feeling victimised by the comments that a client was making in emails against Jews. She had Jewish ancestry and found the comments offensive. Somehow the power dynamic became so strong that she felt unable to challenge the comments.

Supervising this and looking at the emails that had been sent the supervisor could see that it was as if underneath the words the client knew that this was impacting on Helen. There were clear issues with power that the client was expressing and there were increasing criticisms of Helen as well. It had started to feel like bullying. The head of service became involved and it was decided that the online counselling would be ended and the client would be invited to a face-to-face session with another counsellor.

Prevent duty

Prevent duty in a university. Every university will have a responsibility to have a Prevent policy and a policy regarding vulnerability to radicalisation and to be implementing this. It is likely that each university will have appointed a prevent coordinator. There is a prevent coordinator allocated for south-west, south-east, north-west and north-east specifically dealing with universities and colleges. It is wrong to assume that all issues under this policy arise from ISIS or such as they may equally come from issues connected with far-right ideology.

At the time of writing the relevant websites for university specific information about Prevent is www.safecampuscommunities.ac.uk. This includes an HE training module which is easy to follow and gives a helpful overview. There is also training for FE at www.preventforfeandtraining.org.uk.

Summary

Planning out how you will set up online supervision in a university setting is the first step to good practice. For the most part, it is likely that counsellors in this setting will still be doing far more face-to-face work so how online supervision is organised is a key issue.

References

Bond, T. (2016). *Ethical Framework for the Counselling Professions.* Lutterworth: BACP.
Bond, T. (2015). *Good Practice in Action 047: Ethical Framework for the Counselling Professions Supplementary Guidance: Working Online.* Lutterworth: BACP.
Great Britain (1998). The Data Protection Act. London: Stationery Office.
Information Commissioners Office (2016). Available online at: www.ico.gov.uk.

Websites

www.preventforfeandtraining.org.uk
www.safecampuscommunities.ac.uk

PART IV

Training and trends

Chapter 19

The last words – training online supervisors and the future

Anne Stokes

In conversation with Jane Hallett, Gill Jones, Maria O'Brien, Chris O'Mahony, and Jan Stiff

As I was framing the structure of the book, I decided that for the final chapter, I would like to use a discussion format similar to one used in another book (Bor & Stokes, 2011). However, here it is a transcript of a live online conversation. I invited a group of people, all have of whom been involved in the diploma in therapeutic online supervision (DOTS), to join me in an online meeting. The majority of this chapter is taken up with the actual transcript of our discussion around training online supervisors and where we see the future of online supervision.

I chose synchronous text for two reasons. The first is that it captures the discussion in the participants' own words. The second is that it has many of the same elements as a group supervision session, so highlights another aspect of online supervision. We all know each other well, so there is acceptance of teasing and sometimes interrupting each other which would be less apparent in a newer or more formal group. I have deliberately kept some of these parts in the transcript.

Before the meeting I sent the participants the following agenda:

Starting points

- Is it necessary to train specifically as an online supervisor?
- Does that training have to be online?
- What should the training cover?
- How should we train counsellors to use online supervision?
- Experiences as students, tutors and supervisors in training online supervisors
- How do we see online supervision evolving and therefore training needs?
- Anything else.

Inevitably I have had to edit the transcript, not because of content, but simply because it was too long! It was a hard task as the participants had so many useful points to put forward. I have also edited out some but not all of the "typos'" to make it easier to read. Chris O'Mahony, who was a student on the first cohort of

DOTS and a tutor on a later one, was unable to be present and kindly agreed to read the transcript and provide process comments. I have inserted those within the text in brackets.

There are a couple of abbreviations that we often use, but which may be unfamiliar to readers. Sup/ees is shorthand for supervisees and sup/ors for supervisors. DOTS, which is referred to a number of times, is our shorthand for the diploma in online therapeutic supervision.

If you are not used to online meetings, you may find the transcript difficult to read initially, but I hope that you will soon get into the swing. You'll probably notice how much we use each other's names. This highlights who we are addressing our comment to, as we cannot be seen looking at the individual.

Reflective questions

As you read the transcript below, you might like to reflect on:

* what mental images you have of the participants?
* what contributes to these (ethnicity of names, your own association with the names, what group members are saying etc.)?
* how might your mental images change if you heard the voices or met them f2f?
* how your interactions might change if you heard and saw them?

The meeting

Anne Stokes:	Hello everyone I have a hope that we are all here now – early – wonderful!
Gill Jones:	Hi everyone
Anne Stokes:	Can you just say hello, so I know!
[Chris O'Mahony:	Anne demonstrates the importance of checking in with people – they may appear as "online" on Skype, but until they communicate with you directly, it's hard to know if they are really there.]
Jan Stiff:	Afternoon – lovely to be here :)
Anne Stokes:	It's good to "see" you Jan!
Anne Stokes:	Jane – are you here? You are showing as being so.
Gill Jones:	Is Jane with us?
Anne Stokes:	Hmmm – she is added, but her "sign" shows her as away, so she may not be yet.

Jane Hallett:	Hi everyone
Anne Stokes:	Aha – hi Jane
Gill Jones:	Hi Jane
Anne Stokes:	Whew – we have us all!
Jan Stiff:	Hi Jane ☺
Jane Hallett:	Sorry for delay
Anne Stokes:	No probs Jane, we'd only just got ourselves here
Anne Stokes:	OK – would you like to all begin just by typing what you do. E.g., being a tutor for DOTS, being a supervisor for DOTS and elsewhere, being a DOTS student etc
[Chris O'Mahony:	Although it has taken a few minutes for everyone to arrive in the conversation, once all group participants are there, Anne immediately brings up the purpose of the chat. Online conversations tend to get to the point faster than in-person conversations, possibly because of the additional time and effort involved in typing your thoughts rather than speaking them. This can work well as it does here, between people with established relationships who have come to the conversation for a specific purpose. However, a conversation without the usual pleasantries might feel jarring under other circumstances.]
Jane Hallett:	Supervisor for DOTS
Gill Jones:	I've retired from being an OLT Director and tutor and now have a small private supervision practice. Also a supervisor on DOTS
Jan Stiff:	I have been a student and a tutor for OLT on DOTS and an online supervisor for 2 children's charities offering online counselling. I also provide online supervision privately to counsellors working privately online and face-to-face.
Anne Stokes:	Thanks
Anne Stokes:	I think all of us probably think that training as an online supervisor is necessary but what are the reasons we think this?
Anne Stokes:	So why bother to train?
Jan Stiff:	Interesting phrase "why bother" ...
[Chris O'Mahony:	Text-based online supervision allows us to look closely at the words used by supervisor, supervisee and the client. Here, Jan uses ellipsis to indicate that she is not yet finished typing. It can be helpful to break down long statements into smaller chunks to be sent individually. This avoids other participants being confronted with a "wall of text" that may be difficult to read, and simulates the experience of spoken conversation more closely.]

Jan Stiff:	maybe for some it seems like a "bother" surplus to need?
Gill Jones:	I feel more comfortable offering supervision to online counsellors if I've experienced and have some understanding of the medium in which it's delivered.
Gill Jones:	I believe technology strongly influences online sessions and would want to understand why this is.
Jan Stiff:	I totally agree Gill …
Jan Stiff:	and I have found it surprising how newly qualified online counsellors expect supervision to be via video rather than mirroring the medium they use – i.e. IM
Jane Hallett:	I too agree about the influence of technology
Gill Jones:	And I think my understanding needs to come from a "more experienced" point of view than my personal experience.
Anne Stokes:	OK I am going to be the doubter for a moment….
Anne Stokes:	"But if I am trained to work online as a counsellor, why should I then do more training to be an online supervisor? Feels like training organisations are just out to make money from me"
Jan Stiff:	Ohh good one Anne as I think many people feel this …
Jan Stiff:	from personal experience I have seen how vital an experienced online supervisor can be to my practice and that of my supervisees
Jan Stiff:	saying that, they might not have had formal online supervision training – but come with a good amount of expertise and knowledge and experience
Gill Jones:	Is the same case to be made for training to offer supervision whether f2f or online – why do we think it's necessary?
Anne Stokes:	I guess it would be the same question, Gill.
Gill Jones:	Personally I never realised the importance of training for supervision until I appreciated that supervision was a "shared fantasy"
Anne Stokes:	OK – being even more awkward then – if I am a f2f supervisor – fully trained – why can't I just offer online supervision?
Jane Hallett:	I think there is some truth in your devil's advocate comment Anne. Understanding of the technology and its strengths and weaknesses in communicating accurately is vital. So training as online counsellor is vital.
Jan Stiff:	For me, I also wonder about the importance of having a supervisor who has the same/or more knowledge and experience re the specialty you work in e.g., bereavement, CYP, couples counselling – what is more important the speciality or the fact that the supervisor has online training

Gill Jones:	We all seem to agree that training is necessary for online counselling – I have had personal experience of trying to explain email counselling to my (then) f2f supervisor. If the platform isn't fully understood by them, how can we trust our supervisor to 'hold' our concerns as counsellors?
Jan Stiff:	I agree with that Gill ...
Jan Stiff:	and I have come across a number of supervisees ...
Jane Hallett:	However experience as a supervisor of both online and F2F may be sufficient to work as supervisor online if the individual has trained as a F2F supervisor.
Jan Stiff:	and are suffering from vicarious trauma ...
Jan Stiff:	one had to take time off ...
Jan Stiff:	I believe that good online supervision can prevent this helping the counsellor spot the signs at the early stages
[Chris O'Mahony:	Here, a number of conversational threads overlap. Overlapping conversations can happen for many reasons, such as when there are multiple conversations going on between subgroups within the group. They can also happen when turn-taking conversational behaviour (Sacks, et al, 1974) breaks down temporarily, which can be due to group participants having different typing and processing speeds, and the group having difficulty gauging their reaction times without any visual cues. Some groups detail their policy on turn-taking in their ground rules, but these periods of overlapping conversation often resolve themselves spontaneously.

These overlapping conversations can feel chaotic for novices, as there are no visual cues to indicate who is talking to each other. Suler (1997) asserts that if you are plunged into an online conversation, you are likely to "consciously and unconsciously set up mental filters and points of focus that help you screen out 'noise' and zoom in your concentration on particular people or topics of discussion. Often, you become immersed in one or two strings of dialogue and filter out the others". Suler also says that following the conversation is likely to be easier when you are reading along in real time.] |
| **Anne Stokes:** | Jane, I know that both you and Gill have been the group supervisors on DOTS where we train online supervisors. All of the participants were trained online counsellors. I wonder if you were aware of any "things" which might have not arisen if they hadn't first trained as online counsellors. Badly worded but am I clear enough? |

Anne Stokes:	(I am also aware that you, Gill and I were initially barefoot online supervisors till we were able to devise a pilot then a diploma course to train others! So what made me/us believe it was necessary?)
[Chris O'Mahony:	Here, Anne uses another convention that is understood by the group – a statement in brackets is said as an aside to the general conversation, the text equivalent of a whisper.
	Participants may also put actions in brackets, for example (smiling), (cringing), (running away), (jumping up and down).]
Jane Hallett:	stuff the students have shared which wouldn't have arisen if they'd not trained online first
Gill Jones:	I'm not sure if there were any things that could have been lacking in the scenario you present, Anne, but I do think they may not have been made aware of some of the possibilities of the online supervision platform – e.g., using both text and webcam simultaneously in the session?
Gill Jones:	I think the supervision space can be a "play space" to try things out
[Chris O'Mahony:	Throughout the transcript, inverted commas are used around phrases that the group members want to emphasise, serving the same purpose as stressing certain words and syllables when speaking aloud.]
Jane Hallett:	I agree there Gill
Anne Stokes:	Anything else that they might not have been aware of/spotted etc.?
Jan Stiff:	The words "being unconsciously incompetent" come to mind
Anne Stokes:	Say more Jan
Jan Stiff:	I have seen how online counsellors are often surprised by what they "need" to know and what they felt they knew but didn't – hope that makes sense ...
Jan Stiff:	so untrained supervisors could think they were competent enough but might practice unsafely, unethically, poor boundaries etc.
Anne Stokes:	Good point and so I am adding to this. We need to have sup courses to enable practitioners to be competent and confident to offer this to their supervisees?
Gill Jones:	Agree with that, Anne
Gill Jones:	And to explore how to use the space that technology offers
Jane Hallett:	Unconscious incompetence brings a student who I experienced as overconfident to mind.
Jan Stiff:	the training is something to measure their competence by at the beginning and the end – students might come with varying amounts of experience to share with each other too

Jane Hallett:	I like the measure of competence Jan
Anne Stokes:	I guess I also think that the training will hopefully enable even f2f supervisors, who are trained online counsellors, to think about what their online supervision model is – the same, different or tweaked from their f2f model
Gill Jones:	I agree with the enriching process a training course group can offer
Anne Stokes:	Back to your point Jane – so a f2f supervisor may be overconfident in being able to simply set up as an online supervisor?
Jan Stiff:	I see how models can help students develop and believe in a way of supervising online that suits them – hopefully this ensures they are confident in their practice too
Jan Stiff:	(sorry butted in there :))
Jane Hallett:	Very likely of anyone over confident.
Anne Stokes:	NO probs Jan. I will edit as necessary to make it flow more, but this is the reality of an online group conversation
Gill Jones:	Which an online supervisor needs to be able to appreciate and use to their supervisee's advantage ☺
[Chris O'Mahony:	Smileys or emoticons are often used in text conversations to communicate something of the group participant's emotional state or intent to others. They can be used to convey that the preceding statement was meant humorously or light-heartedly, or can indicate irony or sarcasm. Smileys can lessen the ambiguity of text-based conversation, lowering the chances of misunderstanding.]
Gill Jones:	sorry I can't get skype to accept a plural for supervisee
Jan Stiff:	lol ☺
[Chris O'Mahony:	Lol – laugh out oud – is an acronym commonly used online. Different generations and different online communities may have developed different acronyms and internet slang. As a supervisor, you may wish to think about how you would respond to someone you were supervising who used a slang term or acronym that you were not familiar with.]
Jan Stiff:	I find the need for reassurance in much of my own sup of sup and for counsellors I supervise ...
Jan Stiff:	this needs a supervisor who you can trust and feel is proficient
Jan Stiff:	and who understands the complexities of online clients
Jane Hallett:	Agree with both your points Jan
	*** Jane Hallett has left ***
[Chris O'Mahony:	Technical issues can arise in online session. It can be helpful to have a backup plan in case of technological failure.]

Anne Stokes:	OK – so training is about demonstrating competence to our sup/ees/ their clients/ our professional bodies?
[Chris O'Mahony:	Anne is checking back in to make sure she's understood what the other group participants have said – in an online conversation, where we're trying to hear what a person means using just the written word, we may project our own meanings onto others. It's important to check in, perhaps more than we would be face-to-face, to make sure we understand each other.]
Anne Stokes:	Oh Jane has gone. I will try bringing her back in.
Jan Stiff:	definitely
Gill Jones:	and understands where you're coming from, Jan – back to the platforms argument, I think. The technology platforms can enrich sessions so much
	*** Anne Stokes added Jane Hallett ***
Jane Hallett:	Thanks Anne. Using smart phone don't know what I did I☺
[Chris O'Mahony:	This is the first time we hear what kind of technology a group member is using to access the meeting. We don't know where they are, if it's public or private, if others can see what they're doing, if friends or family members are in the same room, if there are a lot of distractions or if it might be an unsafe environment – when conducting online supervision sessions, you may wish to check with your supervisee to determine if their environment is appropriate for supervision at that time.]
Jan Stiff:	this brings tech to light as you say Gill – how does a simple issue such as a client disappearing leave a counsellor feeling.... . is it important for them to explore this
[Chris O'Mahony:	If this happens in online supervision – Jane losing connection to the group – it might parallel an experience in the online counselling relationship that is being reflected upon. Experiencing this in online supervision can help the supervisee to work through the technical side of what to do if this happens in a counselling session, but the experience may also help to work through ways to process the emotional effects on both parties.]
Anne Stokes:	Gill that brings me to another question which I think you have begun to answer. . . . .
Anne Stokes:	if we think that training is necessary for online supervisors.... .
Anne Stokes:	does it have to take place online?
Jan Stiff:	I hear myself shout YES definitely
Anne Stokes:	Why?
Jan Stiff:	could in part be face to face

Jan Stiff:	The more sterile side of theory could be face to face or working alone
Anne Stokes:	LOL Jan – sterile side of theory!!
Jan Stiff:	lol – that's me and theory for you – essential I know but I don't love it!
Gill Jones:	Yes, I agree, Jan – the experiential route for learning has always been my preference and to have things like clients or sup/ees disappearing is a good example
Jane Hallett:	Agree that needs to be explored. Part of restorative sup.
Jan Stiff:	even in role play ...
Jan Stiff:	students experience lapses in contact ...
Jan Stiff:	find this frustrating ...
Jan Stiff:	and might think simply of the other student in the role play but in reality it is valuable learning
Anne Stokes:	actually having teased you, Jan, I am not sure I agree with you. I wonder if in fact the drier theory might be less sterile when taught online in a group. Just thinking about some of the wonderful online sessions DOTS students have run
Jan Stiff:	I agree Anne – have to admit – I would find theory something I avoided if I was set to task it alone – so many benefits of group learning AND sometimes the theory is not 100% correct!
Jan Stiff:	online sup is still at an early stage of development
Jane Hallett:	I think experiential learning vital too. I don't have sufficient evidence but I suspect there is less experiential learning in F2F courses
Anne Stokes:	Oh that is an interesting thought, Jane.
Gill Jones:	We can offer a closer approximation to reality if we offer online experiential training for online supervision
Jan Stiff:	issues of transference and countertransference are also important issues to experience online
Anne Stokes:	So are we saying that ideally online supervision training should be in online courses, and at the very least it needs to be at least partly online?
Jan Stiff:	yes
Jane Hallett:	Agree
Gill Jones:	Yes – I would veer towards courses delivered 100% online myself
Jan Stiff:	there is only a small amount that really can be taught face to face
Gill Jones:	So 90% online Jan?

Jan Stiff:	lol yes
Anne Stokes:	OK – I am tempted to bring Maria in at this point as I can see her online, and I'd be interested to hear what everyone thinks should be in an online supervision training course. She like you, Jan has been a student, and is a tutor now. Would that be OK?
Jan Stiff:	yes ☺
Gill Jones:	Fine by me
Jane Hallett:	Ditto
	*** Anne Stokes added Maria O'Brien ***
Jan Stiff:	Can I add a point whilst we are waiting?
Anne Stokes:	Hi Maria – I saw that you are back and you said you might be able to join us
Maria O'Brien:	Hi, I didn't want to interrupt so I'll just sit quietly.
Anne Stokes:	Go ahead Jan
Jan Stiff:	just to say ...
Jan Stiff:	what suddenly struck me ...
Jan Stiff:	was the issue of working online and how vulnerable and isolated that can leave a practitioner feeling ...
Jan Stiff:	training and group sharing is beneficial here
Jan Stiff:	(done! Hi Maria)
Maria O'Brien:	Hi Jan
Anne Stokes:	Totally agree Jan. So what should be included in an online supervision course?
Gill Jones:	online training in groups can be very supportive after the training ends
Jan Stiff:	yes students often build strong bonds
Jan Stiff:	actually that is another point – supervising in online groups and individually ...
Jan Stiff:	noticing the different needs
Jane Hallett:	The need to develop bonds with colleagues when working online
Jan Stiff:	group dynamics can be a real challenge
Jan Stiff:	and interesting too
Anne Stokes:	So online group dynamics could be a part of the curriculum?
Jan Stiff:	Yes and how disinhibition often works in online groups too
Anne Stokes:	OK – and what else goes in to the curriculum? (Anyone)
Jane Hallett:	Strongly agree re dynamics
Jan Stiff:	Transference and countertransference (just thinking out loud now)
Maria O'Brien:	I would agree with that point Jane

Jane Hallett:	Or specific course to look at dynamics.
Jan Stiff:	Assessment – online counsellors at different stages of development
Jan Stiff:	Supervising for organisations – online
Jan Stiff:	contracting
Jane Hallett:	Contracting BIG YES.
Maria O'Brien:	Thinking about how one would develop a course for group Dynamics.
Gill Jones:	Are we making a good case for an evolving online curriculum for training on ine supervisors?
Maria O'Brien:	Sounds like it.
Anne Stokes:	what would you want in, Gill?
Gill Jones:	All the above –
Gill Jones:	plus a good grounding in how to get the best out of technology
Jan Stiff:	Online relationship – understanding oneself as a practitioner – what limits you
Jan Stiff:	yes Gill I agree ...
Anne Stokes:	(how) is that different from training as an online counsellor, Jan
Jan Stiff:	this can be the biggest stress for me when providing online sup!!
Jan Stiff:	thinking....
Jan Stiff:	there is a different sense of responsibility ...
Jan Stiff:	the triad of the client, the counsellor, oneself and maybe an organisation?
Anne Stokes:	that makes sense
Jan Stiff:	a lot to feel responsible for hence the significance of sup of sup too
Jane Hallett:	I think there is a need for means of keeping up to date with technology. I struggle to do so.
Anne Stokes:	me too
Gill Jones:	Agree Jane, technology is changing all the time and online training should be as up to date as possible. It's a big ask sometimes.
Jan Stiff:	wondering if we need a way to update ourselves in our tech ability
Jane Hallett:	That's what I'm suggesting Jan
Anne Stokes:	just thinking here ... it feels as if quite a bit of what we are saying needs to be in is also applicable to online counsellor training, but somehow the depth and responsibility is different. Maybe also we are modelling for our supervisees.
Maria O'Brien:	Interestingly I notice my response to that being mixed.

Anne Stokes:	Go ahead Maria
Maria O'Brien:	I'll start by reminding you all that it took me a year to find the reply all button on the email program......
Gill Jones:	☺ Maria
Jan Stiff:	Think we have all had similar moments Maria ☺
Maria O'Brien:	In that situation what helped was not someone telling me how to do it but being patient enough to wait until I found my path......
Maria O'Brien:	My understanding of Online supervision is that it's mainly about developing a relationship with the supervisee....
Jane Hallett:	Agree Maria
Maria O'Brien:	For me that means working with wherever they are technology wise......
Jan Stiff:	yes absolutely agree – the relationship is key
Maria O'Brien:	that said...I do see there is a place for keeping up to date with technology.
Jane Hallett:	I am aware however that my technical knowledge limits me.
Gill Jones:	Guess it depends whether the sup/ee is working online or f2f to for me
Maria O'Brien:	When I said to stay with the supervisee I meant in a technological sense.
Anne Stokes:	so may be an "and/and"? We as supervisors may need to be up to date with technology
Jan Stiff:	yes....
Maria O'Brien:	Exactly
Jan Stiff:	and how they might be limited ...
Gill Jones:	agree with you Anne
Maria O'Brien:	And also how our speed may limit them
Jan Stiff:	some work with a VSee platform ...
Jan Stiff:	and tell me how this affects their communication – not having a cursor ...
Anne Stokes:	say more Jan
Jan Stiff:	they feel very limited without a cursor ...
Gill Jones:	Cursor Jan?
Jan Stiff:	it leaves their minds, understandably, open to many thoughts ...
Anne Stokes:	do you mean being able to see whether the person is typing or not?
[Chris O'Mahony:	When using some platforms, it is possible to know that someone is typing a response even though their words are

not appearing on the screen. This happens either through a sentence such as "Anne is typing" or a moving pencil symbol appearing below the chat screen.]

Jan Stiff:	are they bored, are they there etc
Jan Stiff:	yes – sorry
Jan Stiff:	how long do you keep the silence for (maintain)
Anne Stokes:	So VSee may be a safer platform, but has drawbacks which e.g., Skype doesn't?
Jan Stiff:	yes
Anne Stokes:	I am aware of time and that you may all be longing to do other things, but there is another area that I'd just like to touch on if you have time. . . . . .
Jan Stiff:	no problem
Anne Stokes:	that is: how do you see online supervision evolving or indeed-do you see it evolving?
Jan Stiff:	I see online therapists understanding the significance of it evolving
Maria O'Brien:	I see f2f practitioners utilising it more.
Jane Hallett:	I think technological developments may mean online sup evolves.
Jane Hallett:	Using both online and F2F may become more common.
Jane Hallett:	With the one person that is
Gill Jones:	Agree Jane – technology will change and online supervisors need to be aware of the changes – their clients may expect them to work in new platforms
Maria O'Brien:	I think so
Jan Stiff:	understanding the intricacies and issues relating to using video will evolve ...
Jan Stiff:	I think this still needs improved understanding
Jan Stiff:	Hopefully this book itself will help promote the significance of training for online supervision
Anne Stokes:	that is one of my hopes, Jan. If so, it's worth the blood sweat and tears!
Jan Stiff:	We can't all be mad in thinking training is important ☺
Jan Stiff:	yes to those blood sweat and tears – got the t shirt!!
Anne Stokes:	well, we can all be mad and it still be true that training is important.
Maria O'Brien:	And training can be fun
Jan Stiff:	so true Maria – it often is

Maria O'Brien:	Sometimes I forget that.
Gill Jones:	Training is the playground where we can practise our skills
Anne Stokes:	In ending this conversation, does anyone want to share hi-lights and lo-lights from your experiences as students, tutors and supervisors on online supervision courses?
Jane Hallett:	The fun aspect is worth promoting more perhaps
Anne Stokes:	yes Jane!
Maria O'Brien:	I totally agree Jane
Jan Stiff:	I love what Gill has just said – I think that says it all – it gives permission to learn in your own way – there are often no rights or wrongs after all
Gill Jones:	Thanks Jan – didn't realise it was as profound as you've made it.
Jan Stiff:	☺
Jane Hallett:	Low light feeling insufficiently informed to comment on dynamics. Highlight working with Maria last year. Yes I am a creep ☺
Maria O'Brien:	:D
[Chris O'Mahony:	This emoticon cannot be reproduced here as it appears on the screen. It is a symbol for a smile with a large grinning mouth. It does demonstrate that keystrokes can be used to replicate emoticons in some cases within word documents. It is necessary however to check that these are understood by the receiver.]
Maria O'Brien:	I enjoyed it as much as you did Jane.
Gill Jones:	Highlight has been sessions with people who are both knowledgeable and eager to learn more – so often student comments took things forward in unexpected ways
Maria O'Brien:	Highlight has been containing supervisees who didn't believe in themselves.
Anne Stokes:	I think this should make an interesting chapter! Thank you all – I knew you'd all come up with some goodies! The next step is to send it to Chris, who is not able to be here and she may add comments. Then I will edit and send it to all of you. Actually the first thing is to save it! Could others do the same, so if I have a bad tech moment, we do have a record of it!
Jan Stiff:	and all those moments – like now – when I sit back and realise I have been looking at a computer screen for hours – if you didn't know better – it might seem as if I was doing very little where SO much can be achieved training online

Jan Stiff:	(will save too)
Anne Stokes:	I hope you have been getting up every 20 mins, Jan and stretched etc.!
Jan Stiff:	that's another one – no I haven't and rarely do :)
Anne Stokes:	I am very very grateful for this time. I wanted a chapter on training and I think in some ways this demonstrates how group supervision works too. Sort of // process
[Chris O'Mahony:	//in this context is shorthand for parallel.]
Jan Stiff:	I've enjoyed this Anne – it's been really interesting
Jan Stiff:	Good to "see" everyone too
Maria O'Brien:	Yes it's lovely to catch up if it's only brief.
Gill Jones:	It's been lovely to get back in touch with everyone after a break in contact.
Jan Stiff:	a chapter in 1 1/2 hours – if only that had been the case! :)
Anne Stokes:	there is just a tad of editing necessary, Jan!
[Chris O'Mahony:	The warmth in these lines is palpable. The group participants have had a real feeling of presence and togetherness.]
Jan Stiff:	Sorry – totally appreciate that Anne ☺
Jane Hallett:	OK I too need to go. Good to speak with you all. If I don't speak before have a relaxing Xmas. ✳
Jan Stiff:	you too Jane
Anne Stokes:	thanks everyone. Bye for now.

Reflective questions

As you reach the end of the transcript, and indeed the end of the book, perhaps ask yourself these reflective questions:

- What, if anything, have you gained from reading this chapter and the other chapters?
- What questions are you left with?
- Where can you find the answers?
- What is your image of yourself now in relation to Online Supervision?

Despite the blood, sweat and tears mentioned in the transcript, we've enjoyed writing this book. We hope you have enjoyed it too and perhaps more importantly, found it useful.

References

Bor, R. & Stokes, A. (2011). *Setting Up in Independent Practice*. Basingstoke: Palgrave Macmillan.

Sacks, H., Schegloff, E. A., & Jefferson, G. (1974). A simplest systematics for the organization of turn-taking for conversation. *Language, 50(4)*: 696–735.

Suler, J. (1997). Psychological dynamics of online synchronous conversations in text-driven chat environments. *The Psychology of Cyberspace*. Available online at: www-usr.rider.edu/~suler/psycyber/texttalk.html.

Glossary

ACTO   Association for Counsellors and Therapists Online.

BACP   British Association for Counselling and Psychotherapy.

Blended supervision   Supervision that takes place through a combination of in-person and online interactions.

Distance supervision   Supervision when supervisor and supervisee are not in the same physical space.

e-supervision   Alternative name for online supervision.

f2f   face-to-face.

IRC   Internet Relay Chat (live text chat) is a platform where people type their words into a shared private chat screen.

in-the-room   Supervisor and supervisee both being physically in the same room at the same time. Another name for f2f.

In-person   An interaction where the two (or more) parties are within the same physical space, e.g. in-person counselling usually takes place in the counselling room.

OCTIA   Online Counsellors and Therapists in Action. The annual conference for Online Therapy organised by ACTO.

Online counselling   Any form of mental health counselling delivered through remote means. For example, videoconferencing, live chat, email and voice.

Online supervision   Any form of mental health supervision delivered through remote means.

Online text-based supervision   Online supervision that takes place through synchronous or asynchronous text. For example, live chat, email, chat rooms, forums or message boards.

Supervision   A specialised form of professional mentoring provided for practitioners responsible for undertaking challenging work with people. Supervision is provided to ensure standards, enhance quality, advance learning, stimulate creativity, and support the sustainability and resilience of the work being undertaken (BACP, 2016).

Webcam   A webcam is a video camera connected to a computer.
UKCP   United Kingdom Council for Psychotherapy.

Reference

BACP (2016). *BACP Register of Counsellors & Psychotherapists: A Registrant's Guide to Supervision*. Lutterworth: BACP.

Index

For Product Safety Concerns and Information please contact our EU
representative GPSR@taylorandfrancis.com
Taylor & Francis Verlag GmbH, Kaufingerstraße 24, 80331 München, Germany

www.ingramcontent.com/pod-product-compliance
Lightning Source LLC
Chambersburg PA
CBHW050347270326
41926CB00016B/3637